Praise for *The Haywire Heart*

"A great resource to learn about warning signs, treatment options, and so on." —*RUNNER'S WORLD*

"A must-read for any dedicated athlete—it examines the symptoms to watch for, what to do about your risks, and how to protect your heart so you can (safely) enjoy sports for the rest of your life." —*TRIATHLETE*

"In the long term, warn the American authors of a new book, extreme exercisers could be setting themselves up for serious consequences." —*THE TIMES* (LONDON)

"The science is well explained—and backed up by color diagrams and a handy glossary. Ultimately, though, this is a hopeful book on a deadly subject." —*EXPERIENCE LIFE*

"Ultrarunners and other endurance athletes should pay attention to the main message of this fascinating book." —*ULTRARUNNING*

"The field of arrhythmias is rather complicated . . . but the authors have found a writing style that is captivating and accessible to the non-medical reader, while retaining much medical detail that will be of interest." —DR. LARRY CRESWELL, ATHLETESHEART.ORG

"Anyone who does intense or long endurance training, especially over many years, should read this book." —ROADBIKERIDER.COM

"Zinn and fellow authors Chris Case and John Mandrola, a cardiac electro-physiologist and cyclist with atrial fibrillation, do a good job of looking at all the angles." —*CANADIAN CYCLING*

"These authors believe that physical exercise is a positive thing, [but] they urge athletes to be realistic about the danger of pushing the limits of your heart." —*TRIATHLON MAGAZINE CANADA*

"*The Haywire Heart* is intensely readable, informative, and necessary reading for anyone who races bicycles. Seriously." —BIKEISTAN.COM

"Until now, coaches and doctors have chalked up heart problems in athletes to 'preexisting conditions,' but the percentage of athletes with life-threatening problems justifies the warnings in *The Haywire Heart*. The book actually shocked me; I know too many of the athletes in the book. *The Haywire Heart* flows and develops like a great novel, but it is not fiction." —GARY NEPTUNE, MOUNTAINEER

"This book could save your life." —THEWASHINGMACHINEPOST.NET

"*The Haywire Heart* does an excellent job of walking the line between alarmism and reality. Where the book really shines is in the case studies of citizen athletes who have seen their lives turned upside down." —*MADISON MAGAZINE*

"If you have been diagnosed with a cardiac condition . . . *The Haywire Heart* will fill in a lot of blanks for you." —*PODIUM CAFÉ*

"I appreciate how the theme of *The Haywire Heart* is 'Let's focus on longevity as the measuring stick of fitness, not necessarily the world record that we're gonna hold.'" —*40+ FITNESS* PODCAST

THE HAYWIRE HEART

How too much exercise
can kill you, and what you can do
to protect your heart

Chris Case
John Mandrola, MD
Lennard Zinn

Outside Books

Outside Books®

1600 Pearl Street 300
Boulder, Colorado 80302 USA

Outside Books is the leading publisher of books on endurance sports. Focused on cycling, triathlon, running, swimming, and nutrition/diet, Outside Books helps athletes achieve their goals of going faster and farther. Preview books and contact us at outsideinc.com/outside-books.

Distributed in the United States and Canada by Ingram Publisher Services

Library of Congress Cataloging-in-Publication Data

Names: Case, Chris, author. | Mandrola, John, author. | Zinn, Lennard, author.
Title: The haywire heart: how too much exercise can kill you, and what you can do to protect your heart / Chris Case, Dr. John Mandrola, and Lennard Zinn.
Description: Boulder, Colorado: VeloPress, [2017] | Includes bibliographical references and index.
Identifiers: LCCN 2016049013 | ISBN 9781937715670 (hardcover with jacket: alk. paper) | ISBN 9781937715885 (paperback)
Subjects: LCSH: Athletes—Diseases. | Heart—Diseases. | Sports—Physiological aspects. | Sports for older people.
Classification: LCC RC1236.H43 C37 2017 | DDC 617.1/027—dc23
LC record available at https://lccn.loc.gov/2016049013

This paper meets the requirements of ANSI/NISO Z39.48-1992 (Permanence of Paper).

Art direction by Vicki Hopewell
Cover design by Kevin Roberson
Cover photographs by 4×6, Technotr, and Avid Creative, Inc./iStock
Illustrations by Charlie Layton
Composition by Jane Raese

Text set in Helvetica Neue and Freight Text
22 / 10   9   8   7   6   5

CONTENTS

ILLUSTRATIONS

PREFACE

CHRIS CASE

The sun shone bright on the upturned Flatirons rock formations above Boulder, Colorado. It was another perfect day in a cycling paradise. Lennard Zinn, a world-renowned technical cycling guru, founder of Zinn Cycles, author of *Zinn and the Art of Road Bike Maintenance,* longtime member of the *VeloNews* magazine staff, and former member of the US national cycling team, was riding hard up his beloved Flagstaff Mountain, a popular road that snakes over 4 miles and almost 2,000 feet above the city. It was a ride he had done a thousand times before. But on this day, in July 2013, his life would change forever.

Fifteen minutes into his attempt to set a new Strava "king of the mountain" (KOM) time for the climb in the 55-plus age group, he felt his heart "skip" a beat. It was something he had felt before, but only at rest. He looked down at the Garmin computer on his handlebars and noticed that his heart rate had jumped from 155 to 218 beats per minute (bpm) and stayed elevated. He tapped the Garmin's screen. Was the connection bad? He felt fine but eventually pulled the plug on the attempt, knowing that the distraction had disrupted any chance at a record.

His heart rate immediately dropped, so he headed down the mountain to establish a different Strava segment KOM. His training plan called for a very hard ride, so he went to another climb and did a set of intervals. His ride completed, he headed home.

Later that day, he called his physician as a precaution. Much to his surprise, after describing the incident, he was told to head to the emergency room immediately. Then things took an even more serious turn: After a series of tests, the ER physician recommended that he be taken via ambulance to the main cardiac unit of the Boulder hospital for an overnight evaluation.

Despite the initial alarm, his doctors simply prescribed rest. That seemed easy enough. So easy, in fact, that even though he trusted the cardiologists and the ER doctor, he ignored the true depth of their warnings. While he obeyed their calls for rest for a short time, he eventually returned to his usual training plan. His only concession was that he did not resist when he was asked to wear a portable telemetric electrocardiogram (ECG) unit that dangled around his neck (a device known as a Holter monitor); it didn't disrupt his routine.

What did disturb life and training were the annoying episodes that started to become more frequent during his intense rides. Now when his heart rate spiked, he experienced what felt like a flopping fish in his chest.

More upsetting was the phone call in the middle of the night from a faraway nurse who had been monitoring the ECG readings from his

Holter monitor. She had some shocking news: His heart had stopped for a few seconds. He had to finally admit that something was definitely wrong.

By October, Zinn could do nothing to eliminate the episodes. He made every attempt to reduce the stress in his life, but intense riding and racing always triggered an episode of elevated heart rate and that fish-out-of-water feeling. After further visits to his cardiac electrophysiologist, he received an official diagnosis: multifocal atrial tachycardia.

That's when Zinn ultimately decided to heed the warning he'd been given and quit racing. He also backed off from riding with intensity or duration. In doing so, he felt instantaneously downgraded from thoroughbred to invalid. He altered the very nature of his life, in more ways than one. He was made to face the reality that he could never do what he used to do in the same way that he used to do it. He now became interested in maintaining an activity level to sustain his longevity rather than his fitness or speed.

Life had changed. Forever.

Zinn quickly realized he was not alone. When he began the psychologically arduous process of coming to terms with his life-changing condition, he reached out to friends who had been fabulous athletes in their day and who continued to push themselves well into their 40s and 50s.

The number of friends, colleagues, and former teammates who had had similar or more severe heart issues was alarming. Far from being an outlier, Zinn was one among many.

That's when I, as the managing editor of *VeloNews* and a friend and colleague of Zinn, couldn't help but think there was more to this issue than an isolated incident on an iconic climb in a cycling-crazed town. Once I

heard the various stories of heart arrhythmias in masters endurance athletes and read the research literature on the subject, it was obvious that
this would make for a compelling and important article in the magazine.
(An arrhythmia is an irregular heart rhythm caused by a malfunction in
the heart's electrical system. Zinn's tachycardia is but one example.)

With the help of many, particularly Dr. John Mandrola, we published
"Cycling to Extremes: Are Endurance Athletes Hurting Their Hearts by
Repeatedly Pushing Beyond What Is Normal?" in our August 2015 issue.
Mandrola's assistance was critical, as he is a cardiac electrophysiologist
from Louisville, Kentucky, who frequently writes and lectures on the very
subject of endurance athletes and heart health. He has also been a competitive athlete much of his life and has an arrhythmia himself (atrial
fibrillation, which is defined as a rapid and irregular heartbeat above 300
beats per minute).

The response from readers and members of the media was staggering. Zinn, in particular, was inundated by letters, e-mails, and phone calls
from friends, colleagues, and strangers. The overwhelming majority of the
attention came from individuals for whom the article was extremely moving or meaningful, something they could relate to, a story that touched
them unlike anything they had read before. In more than one case, the
article changed a life.

There were also some naysayers, to be sure, those who doubted the connection or took offense at the representation of their cherished pastime and
of exercise in general. It is true that the scientific community is not fully in
agreement on the numerous complex issues involved in heart arrhythmias
and the potential causal connection to lifelong endurance exercise.

Therein lies the very reason for this book. The topic is broad, multifaceted, complicated, and, in so many ways, extremely important to investigate further. Another magazine article wouldn't move the needle very far. We needed a more thorough exploration. Why now? The explosion in popularity of endurance sports has coincided with the ability and desire of an active populace to strive for elite athletic achievements deep into their lives.

Of course, that begs the question: Is exercise good for your heart? Undoubtedly, it is. In fact, it is undeniably the best medicine there is for preventing a host of cardiovascular diseases, as well as a multitude of other diseases. Its documented beneficial results would qualify it as a miracle drug if a pharmaceutical company could figure out how to bottle it. But even miracle drugs have a recommended dosage, and vastly exceeding it is not generally prudent.

Can there be too much of a good thing? Quite possibly—as you'll soon learn. Are endurance athletes hurting their hearts by repeatedly pushing beyond what is normal? Just maybe, and there is a sad and tragic irony to the paradox that those at the highest level of performance could be beset by similar types of heart disease that afflict those who are sedentary or obese, or who smoke. But our hope is that such side effects of an active lifestyle can be prevented with a better understanding of exercise and heart health.

After reading this book, you'll have that understanding of how and why endurance sports could damage your heart. We'll review the evidence, which has been aided in recent years by advancements in research techniques such as magnetic resonance imaging and a more robust understanding of genetics, all of which has helped inform researchers as to the mechanisms that cause damage. If you're an athlete (or have one in your family), you will acquire the necessary tools to make more informed decisions about what is an appropriate amount of training. For those who suspect they may have an arrhythmia or are feeling cardiac symptoms, we will guide you on what to do next. You'll read real-life case studies of exercise-induced disease.

In short, you'll understand a problem that until now has often included more lore than fact. And for those of you who have already developed an arrhythmia, perhaps this book can bring you comfort in knowing that you're not alone, and that life does not have to end. There can be a rich and rewarding life on the other side of your diagnosis, if you are patient, well-informed, and persistent.

Introduction

CHRIS CASE AND JOHN MANDROLA

FOR THE PAST FEW YEARS, a debate about whether too much exercise can be bad for your health has been playing out in popular media. Maybe you've seen some of the articles—they've appeared in the *New York Times, Sports Illustrated,* the *Wall Street Journal, U.S. News and World Report,* and many other places. With titles like "The Great Fitness Debate: Is It True That You Can Exercise Too Much?" and "Can Too Much Exercise Harm the Heart?" they instantly grab the attention of many readers. After all, we've been told for decades that exercise is the best medicine for your heart. Now there's a chance it's harmful? What is a person to believe?

Sometimes the authors of these articles pit one camp against another, stating things like "the too-much-exercise advocates believe. . .," as if this were a political debate, with one side being right and the other side being misinformed at best and dangerous at worst. Occasionally the authors

1

suggest that those who believe there can be too much exercise are verging on alarmism. (Let us emphasize that the authors of this book are anything but alarmists. In fact, all three are lifelong endurance athletes with a penchant for riding hard and suffering often. That is, until two of them were made to slow down after developing heart arrhythmias, which you'll soon learn more about.)

Some authors may cite studies that look at Olympians or professional cyclists who've competed in the Tour de France and find no lasting negative effects on the heart. Are you an Olympian? Have you ever raced in the Tour de France? Could it be that the athletes who have reached such heights in sports are genetically different from you and me? Maybe they're not the best examples for understanding what is happening in the hearts of the general population. (There's also the fact that Olympians and professional cyclists tend to relax after they've retired, more often than not. It's just the middle-aged people who *think* they're training to race the Tour who can't seem to stop themselves from pushing so hard for so long.)

As you can see by holding this book in your hands, this is a topic massive in scope and complexity, without simple answers. Almost nothing about this subject is black and white. There's a good chance the aforementioned articles suffer from oversimplification. That's not to say this book has all the answers, either. Far from it. Much more research is needed to settle the issue of just how much exercise is safe, and to better understand the links between exercise dosage and heart health. Scientific research in this area not only is relatively new but is hard to conduct given the limited number of people who fall into the mold of the longtime endurance athlete.

It cannot be stated enough: Exercise is extremely beneficial for heart health. Dozens of large epidemiological studies have found that people who exercise in any amount, whether five minutes a day or two hours a day, are much less likely to develop or die from heart disease than people who are inactive. (That being said, exercise does not make you immune to every heart problem that exists, especially if you have a history of unhealthy living, eating poorly, or smoking or are genetically predisposed to conditions that affect the heart.) These benefits are especially important in this era. The Western world now suffers from a near epidemic of chronic diseases wrought by the toxic combination of too much food and too little exercise.

No one in the health field doubts that regular exercise promotes and maintains physical, mental, and emotional health. Structured exercise can even be used to treat disease. Examples include cardiac rehabilitation in patients with coronary artery disease and heart failure, and pulmonary rehabilitation for patients with emphysema.

Recently, a group of researchers from Adelaide, Australia, showed that overweight and sedentary patients with a heart arrhythmia called atrial fibrillation who exercised enough to gain fitness ended up with less arrhythmia burden. (Their hearts no longer had as many periods of abnormal heart rhythm.)[1] Exercise in this study behaved like an antiarrhythmic drug.

As we've already observed, if exercise were a marketable pill or procedure, it would be a blockbuster. That's why it's difficult for us to write about the possibility that exercise can be harmful. But there are many studies suggesting just that.

The limits of exercise science

Although the evidence confirming the health benefits of low- to moderate-dose exercise is strong, the science that explores high-dose exercise is much more speculative and controversial.

An important reason is the type of studies used in exercise science. The strongest evidence in all of medicine comes from the blinded randomized controlled trial. In this type of study, one group of individuals is randomly selected to have treatment X and another group gets treatment Y. Randomization is used to even out any differences in the two groups for things like age, gender, and socioeconomic status. In the experiment, researchers strive to make the two treatments the only difference between the two groups in the study. Blinding makes it impossible for anyone to know which treatment was received. That way, if there is a difference in a subject's outcome, it can only be attributed to the treatment.

These sorts of trials are impossible in sports medicine. It's easy to see how a randomized controlled study would never be able to answer the too-much-exercise question. First, athletes cannot be blinded to their exercise exposure. Second, there are many variables that affect the occurrence of heart disease. Things like exercise duration and intensity, other stressors in life (divorce, illness, job), family history, and diet all factor into the development of heart disease.

The lack of controlled trials weakens the evidence base in sports medicine. It means we must rely on less rigorous types of studies. These include observational, mechanistic, and animal studies.

Observational trials are problematic because without randomizing the groups and controlling all the trial's factors, one cannot determine cause and effect. For instance, an observational study could suggest long-term endurance exercise *associates* with heart problems, but it cannot easily say long-term endurance exercise *causes* heart problems.

The reason for this important difference is that when you observe nonrandomized groups, you cannot exclude confounding factors and biases. A common bias is that only athletes with problems seek medical attention; the majority of people who compete could be doing well. This is called selection bias.

Mechanistic studies pose problems because they merely provide a plausible way in which endurance exercise could damage the heart. For instance, we describe studies that show modest increases in the cardiac enzyme troponin in athletes right after finishing a major long-distance race. Troponin is typically released during heart injury (e.g., heart attack). This type of study, therefore, supports the hypothesis that repeated bouts of exercise that are intense enough to release an enzyme associated with heart damage could, over time, lead to heart disease. But it's just a hypothesis—a plausible one, but a hypothesis nonetheless.

Animal studies are limited for obvious reasons: Animals are not people. That doesn't mean animal studies are useless; in fact, they can be quite helpful. But it does mean that they are largely speculative.

As you can see, exercise science faces a few challenges. That doesn't mean the results of the emerging research should be ignored or marginalized as inaccurate or inconsequential. It does mean that it's much harder to prove conclusively that one thing causes another—that high-dose exercise causes heart arrhythmias, for example. Thus, the debates will continue to stir in popular media. And researchers will continue to seek answers.

Exercise dosage

Even the best of things can be overdone: Water and oxygen can be lethal in high enough doses. Too much water leads to hyponatremia (low sodium in the blood), and prolonged exposure to high levels of oxygen can damage lung tissue. The old saying holds true: "everything in moderation." Sometimes, there truly can be too much of a good thing.

As you'll soon see, there is also a growing body of evidence to suggest that long-term endurance exercise can have negative consequences for your heart. Let's be very clear about what we mean by that: We're talking about a highly elevated level of exercise that is not only extremely intense but often competitive and is performed for years, if not decades.

There is little that is "normal" or "regular" about the exercise dosages that we will review. But if you're reading this book, you may very well be one of those "abnormal" folks who partakes in this kind of activity, and may have for decades. You're not alone.

The dose of exercise that promotes health is surprisingly small. A study of more than 13,000 men and women who were followed for eight years showed that although death rates decreased with greater levels of fitness, the largest reduction occurred between the sedentary group and those with low levels of fitness.[2] How low? Mortality benefit in this study plateaued at levels of fitness that represent half of what is expected from a trained athlete.

A larger, more recent study confirmed the plateau effect of exercise. In a 12-year study of Taiwanese subjects, researchers also found lower death rates (both from heart disease and cancer) with increasing levels of daily physical activity, but the degree of benefit lessened after 30–60 minutes of exercise per day.[3]

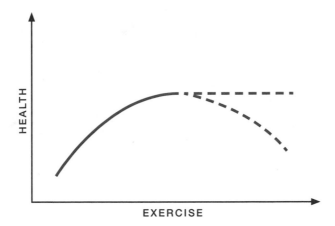

FIGURE I.1. Does more exercise mean greater health? Or is there a point at which too much exercise becomes detrimental?

The take-home message from these findings is that if health is your goal, you need not exercise more than 30–60 minutes each day. Of course, most who participate or compete in endurance sports far exceed these levels of exercise.

The question is, does exercise have an upper-dose benefit limit? Does the health benefit of exercise reverse at higher doses of exercise? Is there a U-shaped curve (Figure I.1)?

These questions and many more will be addressed in Chapter 4, where we'll review the evidence supporting an association between certain types of heart arrhythmias and endurance exercise. Before that, however, let's take a brief look at how the heart works and assess the increased demands placed on the athlete's heart.

1 | How the heart works

LENNARD ZINN

THERE IS ARGUABLY no more important organ in the body than the heart. It is a bit longer and about as wide as an adult fist—about 13 centimeters long and 9 centimeters across. It weighs just over half a pound, or a bit more than that in highly conditioned athletes. If that little muscle, located behind the lower breastbone and slightly to the left of center, were to stop pumping, life would cease in minutes. It is a miracle of plumbing and electrical circuitry, and both have to function properly for it to do its job well.

Plumbing

The heart is actually two pumps in one, with a vertical wall (the septum) separating the left pump from the right pump. (Right and left in cardiac terminology are from the perspective of the heart owner, not from that of an observer facing him or her.) The right side pumps blood to the lungs, and the left side pumps blood to the body.

The heart's four chambers contract in a precisely timed choreography to keep the body supplied with oxygen. The two smaller, upper chambers, called atria (the singular is atrium) or auricles, push blood down to the two larger, lower chambers, called ventricles (Figure 1.1). The heart's right side receives deoxygenated (carbon dioxide–rich) blood from the

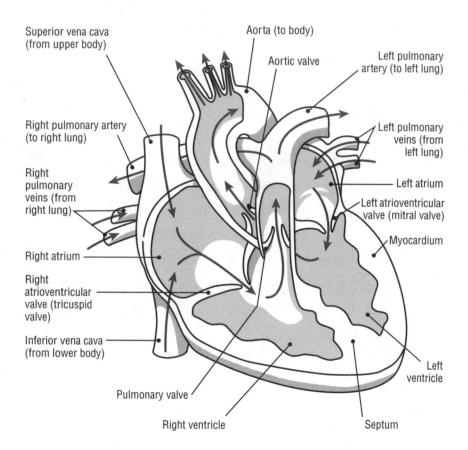

FIGURE 1.1. Cross-section of the heart

body and pumps it to the lungs, and the left side receives oxygenated blood from the lungs and pumps it throughout the remainder of the body. This requires considerable pumping pressure, as the total length of the blood vessels fed by the heart is over 60,000 miles.[1]

Small peripheral veins bring blue blood drained of oxygen from the cells into ever-bigger veins and finally through the two largest return veins, the superior and inferior vena cava, into the right atrium. The atrio-ventricular (AV) valves separating the upper and lower chambers are open when the heart is relaxed (during "diastole"), so the upper atrium passively fills (Figure 1.2). Upon atrial contraction, the right atrium then pushes the rest of this blue blood down into the right ventricle.

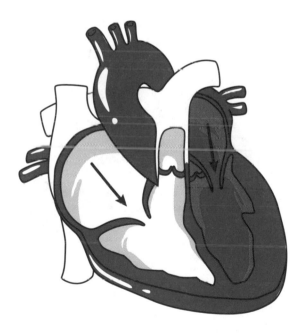

FIGURE 1.2. Cardiac diastole: Chambers are relaxed, blood flows in

As the ventricles begin contracting (the start of "systole"), the tricus-pid valve (the right AV valve) closes to prevent blood from going back up into the right atrium as pressure builds in the ventricle (Figure 1.3). The right ventricle then ejects its full load of blue blood through the open pulmonary valve and into the pulmonary artery to the lungs so it can gather oxygen.

Once the heart is again in diastole (relaxed), red blood full of oxygen flows from the lungs via the four pulmonary veins into the left atrium, and it flows passively into the left ventricle through the open left AV valve (the mitral valve). Then the left atrium contracts, pushing the last of this

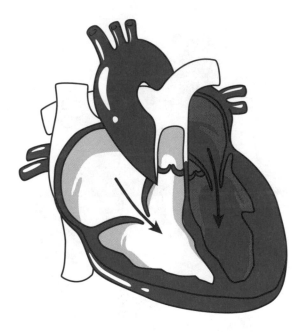

FIGURE 1.3. Atrial systole, ventricular diastole: The atria contract and push blood into the ventricles

red blood down into the left ventricle. The mitral valve closes as the ventricles begin to contract, and the left ventricle's full contraction pushes
that red, oxygen-rich blood through the open aortic valve, into the huge
arch-shaped artery called the aorta, and into the body's vast network of
arteries, literally delivering lifeblood to the body's cells. This completes
one cycle of the heart (Figure 1.4).

This cycle repeats every second or so when the body is at rest, and up
to 3.5 times per second (210 bpm) at high levels of athletic activity. Amaz-
ingly, the heart's four valves open and close passively; the mounting and

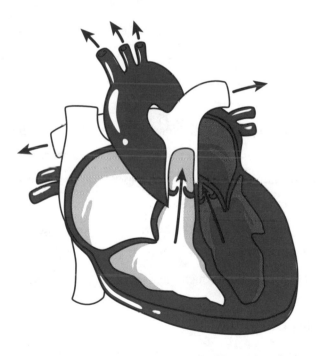

FIGURE 1.4. Atrial diastole, ventricular systole: The atria relax and the
ventricles contract to push blood out of the heart

falling pressure of the blood in the chambers controls the opening and closing of the valves.

The heart's valves open and close precisely so that contractions only send blood in a single direction. That "lub-dub, lub-dub, lub-dub" sound we hear when we place our ear on someone's chest right above the heart is actually the sound of the heart's valves opening and closing. Lub is called S1—the turbulence caused by closure of the mitral and tricuspid valves. Dub is called S2, and it's the sound of the pulmonic and aortic valves closing.

Blood pressure, measured in milligrams of mercury (mm Hg), is the pressure that the blood puts on the walls of the blood vessels. Blood pressure depends on the force of the squeeze, the diameter and tension of the blood vessel walls, and the timing of the aortic valve closure. "Diastolic pressure" is the pressure of the blood against the walls of the vessels when the ventricles are filling with blood (that is, when the heart is relaxed). During the heart's ventricular contraction, the pressure of the blood against the arterial walls increases; this is called "systolic pressure."

Systolic and diastolic blood pressure can be measured with a blood pressure cuff; systolic pressure is the upper number, diastolic pressure the lower. Pulmonary blood pressure can be estimated by echocardiogram, which is a sonogram of the heart using sound waves bounced off the heart. It can also be measured directly with a catheter in the pulmonary artery, often placed through the right side of the heart.

Electrical circuitry

The heart is comprised almost entirely of cardiac muscle cells (myocardium). The heart muscle conducts electricity from cell to cell much like an electrical wire carries current through an appliance. Each squeezing heart muscle cell is also a conduit for electrical control of the heart.

Clustered in discrete places throughout these muscle cells are a number of unique pacemaker cells, called autorhythmic cells, that can spontaneously depolarize momentarily from a negatively charged state to a positively charged state to generate the signal for the heart to contract (doctors say these cells have automaticity). The heart keeps pumping regularly and rhythmically without any outside impetus because heart cells are the only cells in the body that can contract on their own without receiving a signal from the nervous system.

Atop the hierarchy of pacemaker cells are those that comprise the sinoatrial (SA) node, located in the upper portion of the right atrium; that's in the northwest if you're looking at the patient's heart as you would a map (Figure 1.5). The SA node, often called the heart's pacemaker, ordinarily establishes the heart's rhythm, and it modifies the rate at which it generates impulses based on neural or hormonal signals. For example, signals from the "fight-or-flight" sympathetic nerves coming out of the upper thoracic portion of the spine accelerate the heart rate, whereas impulses from the vagus nerve, which runs down the left side of the neck and is part of the calming, parasympathetic nervous system, slow the heart rate. Heart rate varies widely in response to these influences.

When in proper coordination, the heart's rhythmic sequence of contractions is called "sinus rhythm." The SA node, in conjunction with the atrioventricular (AV) node, coordinates this rhythm. Electrical impulses originate at the SA node and course downward (think north to south) to the AV nodal cells, which lie near the center of the heart between the

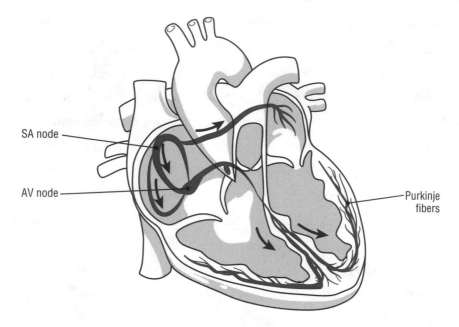

FIGURE 1.5. The heart's electrical circuitry

atria and ventricles and between the left and right sides of the heart. Under normal conditions, the atrial impulse can only get to the ventricle through the AV node, where it gets delayed for 0.1–0.2 seconds. This delay in the node allows the atrial contraction to top up the ventricles, filling them with blood.

Once the signal passes through the AV node, it goes into a specialized conduction system called the "His-Purkinje network," which is the fastest electrical pathway in the heart. Absent a signal from the SA node, the pacemaker cells comprising the AV node can take over the heart's pacemaking, serving as a backup in case the SA node fails for some reason. If both nodes cease to function, other pacemaker cells, including Purkinje fibers, have the ability to initiate electrical signals to keep the heart beating. (These lower subsidiary pacemaker cells frequently save people who develop a block of their SA or AV nodal cells. The rate of the back-up pacemakers is quite low, however; patients with these rhythms feel terrible but they usually survive long enough to get to the doctor.)

The right and left His-Purkinje bundle branches pass down through the right and left ventricles. Once the signal reaches the heart's bottom tip (apex), it spreads out through finer Purkinje fibers, where it then moves up through the heart muscle, coordinating simultaneous right and left ventricular contraction.

The His-Purkinje network is reliable, but like any electrical distribution system, it can be subject to outages. Left bundle branch block (LBBB) is one example: Patients with LBBB have normal conduction of the portion of the impulse intended for the right ventricle through the right bundle, but conduction of the other half of the impulse is impaired; it bypasses the left bundle and must travel through the heart muscle to get to the left ventricle, a slower route. This dyssynchrony means the right ventricle contracts slightly before the left ventricle. Some patients feel this as shortness of breath, and other patients develop compromised heart function from it. Some LBBB patients don't feel any symptoms at all.

Electrical signal propagation

This is where the story gets more complex. If you hated high school biology, no one will blame you for skipping ahead to the next chapter. You won't miss the greater point of the book. If you have a desire to understand the cellular underpinnings of heart arrhythmias, however, please read on.

Skeletal muscles conduct electricity only along their length, since all of the cells in a muscle fiber are fused together and share the same cell membrane. By contrast, cells of the heart can propagate an electric charge to surrounding cells in all directions. So when the electric charge leaves the Purkinje fibers, it travels in a wave throughout the ventricles. The muscular contraction begins squeezing the ventricles from the bottom and continues upward in order to push blood out through the exits of the aorta and the pulmonary artery, both of which are close to where the ventricles and atria meet at the center of the heart (Figure 1.6).

The muscles of the ventricles maintain their contraction until the blood has been pushed out of the exits and the aortic and pulmonary valves close, at which point those ventricle muscles all relax together. Similarly, the atrial contraction also propagates progressively downward from the SA node, with the cells maintaining their contraction until they have squeezed blood out of the upper chambers and into the lower chambers.

Muscle squeezing requires an electrical signal. The signaling occurs by changing the charge of the cell. This "depolarization" of the cells results from the movement of ions in and out of each cell to decrease the relative polarization (i.e., separation) of electric charge on the inside and outside of the cell. Ions are atoms or molecules that carry a net electrical charge, either positive or negative, by virtue of having lost or gained one or more electrons, which carry a single negative charge. Negatively charged ions (anions) have an extra electron or two, whereas positively

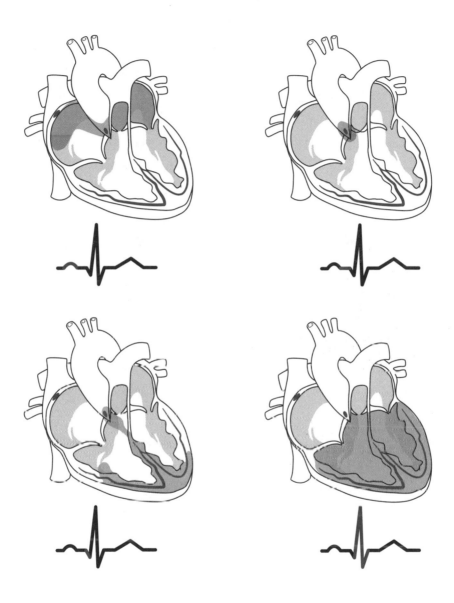

FIGURE 1.6. Electrical signals travel in a wave through the heart. The corresponding portion of the ECG trace is shown below each figure.

charged ions (cations) have lost an electron or two. If free to do so, negatively charged particles will flow from an area of net negative charge toward an area of net positive charge and vice versa; this occurs during depolarization of the cell.

Electrical potential energy (or voltage) is created by polarization, which is simply a spatial separation of oppositely charged ions. Electrical potential energy (often simply called "potential") is the electrical version of mechanical potential energy; if you lift a heavy object, you create mechanical potential energy that will be converted to kinetic energy if you drop it. Cells create electrical potential in a similar way, by concentrating positive charge in one area and negative charge in another.

Each cardiac cell is surrounded by a cell membrane, which is impermeable to charged particles. For a charged particle to move through the cell—to go from inside the cell to outside, let's say—it must pass through a particular kind of hole in the cell wall formed by a cluster of proteins (specifically, a transmembrane protein pore allowing passage of an ion through the membrane). The cell has a number of these pores of different types. A "gap junction" allows charged particles to pass directly from one cardiac cell into another, thus making a string of these cells akin to a wire that can transmit electricity. (Gap junctions conduct in both directions, whereas ion channels usually allow flow only in one direction.) A "voltage-gated ion channel" is another type of pore in the cell membrane; it is regulated by the relative amount of charge on either end of it. Voltage-gated ion channels only allow one-way movement of a certain type of ion through the membrane, and cardiac cells have channels specific to sodium (Na^+), potassium (K^+), calcium (Ca^{2+}), and chloride (Cl^-) ions.

The difference in charge between the inside and outside of the cell membrane is called the "membrane potential" (or "membrane voltage"), which requires energy for the cell to create. The "resting membrane potential" of a muscle cell relative to its surroundings is measured in millivolts (mV; one millivolt is a thousandth of a volt) and is always a negative charge. A cardiac muscle cell maintains a resting potential of about –90 mV by continuously running its sodium-potassium pump, which pushes three sodium (Na^+) ions out of the cell for each two potassium (K^+) ions it pulls into the cell, using up one adenosine triphosphate (ATP) molecule—the unit of energy transfer in the body—in the process.

Think of the transmembrane channels used by the sodium-potassium pump as revolving doors into a hotel lobby; the cell loads up the interior side of the door with three Na^+ cations and the exterior side with two K^+ cations and then spins the door around. And just as when you enter the revolving door with your luggage while somebody on the other side does the same, once the door gets going, there is no going back until you pop out the other side.

Continuously exchanging three Na^+ cations (out) for two K^+ cations (in) not only makes the inside of the cell more negative, but also maintains the concentration of sodium high outside of the cell and low inside, while the opposite condition holds with potassium. In other words, the energy-dependent exchange creates both voltage and concentration gradients so that the cell is ready for depolarization. If it weren't for the impermeability of the cell membrane to ions, the potassium and sodium ions would immediately flow back the other way to neutralize these gradients.

Another cation, calcium (Ca^{2+}), triggers contraction of muscle cells by causing its myofilaments to shorten. So that it can contract when called upon to do so by an electrical signal, a cardiac cell also maintains a calcium gradient internally and externally. It stockpiles Ca^{2+} internally in a compartment called the "sarcoplasmic reticulum," which both stores calcium and, when stimulated, pumps it out into the surrounding sarcoplasm, in which the cell maintains a low calcium concentration between contractions. Like Na^+ levels, Ca^{2+} levels are much higher in the fluid surrounding the cell than in the sarcoplasm within the cell.

When a muscle cell depolarizes, sodium ions pour into it, and some of these ions flow through gap junctions into the surrounding heart muscle cells, slightly depolarizing their membrane potentials and reducing their sodium concentration gradients. Achieving a certain threshold membrane voltage in each of these surrounding heart muscle cells triggers a cascade of opening of their voltage-gated sodium channels, and sodium rushes through them, rapidly depolarizing the cells. Some sodium passes through gap junctions, moving from each of these depolarizing muscle cells into neighboring cells to initiate their depolarization. The cascade continues as the sodium keeps moving through gap junctions into surrounding cells. This process rapidly propagates the electrical signal throughout the cardiac muscle in a wavelike fashion, with each little heart cell contributing action to a muscle that contracts and relaxes.

Muscle-to-muscle conduction is the critical step in electrical coordination of the heart and is an area where much heart rhythm disease occurs, in both atria and ventricles. Earlier we noted that the heart muscle fiber itself conducts like a wire, and that normal heart muscle sends electricity in a smooth wave through the heart. Problems with this conduction appear when areas of the heart muscle become infiltrated with scar tissue, fat, or inflammation. These areas disrupt the smooth wave of electricity much like a boulder in a stream disrupts smooth water flow. The disruption in flow manifests as heart rhythm problems.

Long-term competitive endurance training may cause a scar within the heart muscle. The scar is usually not uniform; there are surviving channels of muscle through it as well as around it. When the smooth wave of electricity approaches the scar, short-circuits can occur. Doctors call these short-circuits "reentry." Reentry due to scarring or other structural disease is a common cause of tachycardia.

The electrical signal to contract

The rate at which sodium depolarizes a cardiac cell is faster than in a skeletal-muscle cell, lasting as little as a millisecond (ms) and rapidly reversing the polarity of the cell from -90 mV to $+50$ mV. This rapid sodium influx into a heart cell triggers the opening of L-type (for "long-lasting") voltage-dependent calcium channels through its cell membrane.[2] Calcium entering the cell through these channels triggers release of yet more calcium from the sarcoplasmic reticulum, causing contraction of the cell.

The squeezing of the heart cell takes time. That's why cardiac muscle has slower calcium channels. After depolarization from the rapid inflow of sodium, calcium then begins moving into the cell through special calcium channels. This slower flow of positive calcium ions keeps the membrane voltage positive for 0.3–0.4 seconds, long enough to contract.

Contraction occurs because the flow of calcium within the cell triggers the release of more calcium from the sarcoplasmic reticulum. Calcium release occurs on a long time scale thanks to a cardiac cell's L-type calcium channels on its membrane. This long-duration calcium release allows heart muscle cells to maintain their contraction for a longer time than skeletal muscle cells. This is critical for efficiently wringing as much blood as possible out of the heart; the contraction not only must squeeze upward through the ventricles from the heart's apex to push blood up and out, but the contraction must also be maintained below so that none of that blood can flow back down as the upper parts of the ventricles contract.

On the voltage-versus-time graph (Figure 1.7) of the cardiac action potential that causes contraction of a cardiac cell, you can see that the slope of the Phase 0 section of the curve corresponding to the influx of

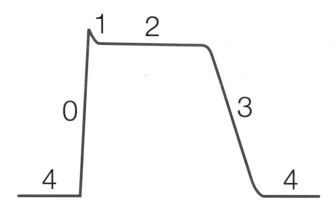

FIGURE 1.7. Action potential (membrane voltage versus time) in a cardiac cell. Phases of the cycle are denoted as 0, 1, 2, 3, or 4.

sodium is almost vertical, indicating how quickly depolarization occurs. Due to its calcium-induced calcium release, the heart cell's action potential has a flat top (Phase 2)—rather than the sharp peak a skeletal-muscle action potential would have—thanks to calcium flowing in over a longer period of time. A small amount of potassium is constantly escaping the cell through potassium leak channels, but when the voltage-gated potassium channels finally cascade open and the sodium and calcium channels close, the cell's membrane potential plummets (Phase 3) to the flat, stable, resting negative level (Phase 4) that the cell maintains between contractions.

If you've ever seen an electrocardiogram, the curve in Figure 1.7 might look vaguely familiar. That's because the spikes and blips on an ECG depict the magnitude and duration of this cellular depolarization.

Pacemaker cells and "skipped beats"

Pacemaker cells activate differently. There is no flat top (Phase 2) to the action potential (Figure 1.8); they don't maintain a contraction. Instead of having a stable resting membrane voltage like other cardiac cells, a pacemaker cell's membrane potential during diastole (when the heart is relaxed) is unstable and gradually depolarizes by allowing sodium ions (primarily) to enter. This shows up in Figure 1.8 as an upslope during the (resting) Phase 4 until it reaches a threshold membrane voltage (the "pacemaker potential") of around –40 mV. When the pacemaker cell hits this threshold potential, it then rapidly depolarizes by the sudden opening of "T"-type (for "transient," meaning fast-acting) voltage-gated calcium channels in its membrane (Phase 0 in the figure).[3]

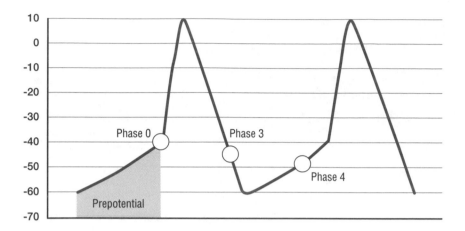

FIGURE 1.8. Action potential (membrane voltage versus time) in a pacemaker cell

When the autonomic nervous system modifies the heart rate, it does so in the SA node, during Phase 4 (the "pacemaker phase"). Stimuli from the sympathetic nerves—fight-or-flight responses—induce increases in heart rate by increasing the slope of the pacemaker phase, thereby decreasing the interval between consecutive pacemaker action potentials. Parasympathetic stimuli (stable, calming influences) from the vagus nerve decrease the slope of Phase 4 in SA nodal cells and lengthen the time between pacemaker action potentials.[4]

The thing is, any cell can get to its pacemaker potential either by gradual, spontaneous depolarization during diastole (resting phase) or by an electrical impulse coming from another pacemaker cell, like the SA node. Since spontaneous depolarization in most of the heart's pacemaker cells happens on a time scale that is slower than the frequency at which signals arrive from the SA node, the SA node generally dictates the heart rate. Spontaneous depolarization happens faster in the SA node than in other pacemaker cells, typically 60 to 100 action potentials per minute (that is, its Phase 4 slope is steeper than in the action potential graph of other pacemaker cells), and it precedes all others in generating electrical impulses.

With conditioning, however, your heart can enlarge and pump significantly more blood with each beat,[5] and your body can use oxygen more efficiently. Accordingly, when at rest, the parasympathetic nervous system recognizes that blood flow is sufficient at a lower heart rate, and it sends signals to the SA node to reduce the rate. Indeed, in some athletes resting heart rate can drop below 30 beats per minute. If the resting rate drops below the rate of spontaneous depolarization of some pacemaker cells, those pacemaker cells can depolarize before a signal to do so comes from the SA node, and this timing disagreement between the SA node and the pacemaker cells will initiate premature heartbeats.

Perhaps you've had the experience, while resting quietly, of your heart feeling like it stopped momentarily. A coach may have told you that you are feeling "skipped beats," and that they are benign and nothing to worry about. In fact, these episodes are generally not missed beats but are actually premature contractions (or "premature complexes"). They feel like skipped beats because the heart chamber contracts out of phase. When this happens, the chamber does not get a chance to fill completely with blood before it contracts, and little or no blood flow results from the contraction. A pause generally follows when the out-of-phase contraction hits the SA node and resets it to its underlying rate (say, 48 bpm at rest), and the SA node then waits its normal time period between contractions before initiating a new heartbeat.

If occurring in the atria, premature contractions are called "premature atrial complexes" (PACs). If they occur in the ventricles, they are called "premature ventricular complexes" (PVCs). Both can be caused by healthy pacemaker cells, but they are more often created by clusters of cells that have somehow gained "enhanced automaticity" and are behaving like pacemaker cells. In the heart of a highly trained athlete, the stimulation from the SA node can be so infrequent that rogue cells behaving as pacemaker cells occasionally fire on their own before the SA nodal cells do.

Similarly, rogue muscle cells in a ventricle can cause PVCs in an athlete's slowly beating heart for the same reason. These PVCs can happen frequently in some elite masters athletes—on the order of 25,000 PVCs per day! That's so disruptive that blood flow is significantly reduced, and treatment—or at least a great reduction in athletic workload—is mandated. We'll discuss premature beats and their treatment options in later chapters.

Fail-safe

Death from fibrillation caused by the disruption of electrical signals can be prevented by the heart's engagement of certain fail-safe modes. The AV node, in particular, has an amazing property in which it slows its conductivity when it becomes stimulated too frequently.[6] This prevents the AV node from sending signals to the ventricles too rapidly if rapid atrial rhythm is occurring, such as during arrhythmic events like atrial fibrillation (AF) or atrial flutter (a more organized and slightly slower rhythm than AF). In essence, the AV node effectively becomes the heart's pacemaker if signals from the SA node become erratic or overly rapid. If the atria go a bit haywire and contract too fast or in an uncoordinated way, the person stays alive as long as the ventricles push whatever blood they can get from the atria out to the lungs and body. But if the ventricles fibrillate, no blood gets to the brain and body, and it's lights out.

Electrical impulses propagate freely between cardiac muscle cells in every direction so that the myocardium functions as a single contractile unit. While this is wonderful for making the heart work efficiently and rapidly, the potential downside of this property is that it can also allow incorrect electrical signals to propagate through the muscle.

The heart's operation is nothing short of miraculous. It's amazing that all of these complex chemical, electrical, and mechanical stimuli and responses occur repeatedly and perfectly, time after time, even at 200 beats per minute or more. And the heart never gets a muscle cramp. It has to relax almost instantaneously after the ventricles have contracted in order to let blood back in to refill them, particularly at high heart rates. And then it needs to start the contraction process all over again.

It's been doing that your entire life. If you're reading this book because you've encountered some heart issues, the following chapters should help you understand what they are, where they come from, and what you can do to address them.

CASE STUDY
Gene Kay: Premature ventricular complexes
Diagnosed at age 54

CHRIS CASE

GENE KAY first got on Nordic skis when he was six years old. He didn't stop racing until he was 54.

During that time, he had a personal goal to do 100 ski marathons. He estimates he racked up 75 of them and many other "marathon" events, including mountain bike races, trail runs, and triathlons. He competed in the elite wave of the Birkebeiner Nordic ski race more than 20 times. He described life as a chronic marathon training session.

When he was 54, all of that changed. After taking a month off following another Birkebeiner, Kay returned to training. Yet he couldn't catch his breath going up stairs. He felt lethargic during his interval sessions. "I could notice it especially at rest," he says. "Sitting around, I could feel like my heart was working quite hard. I'd have one, two, or maybe one, two, three heartbeats and then nothing—there would be a pause and then it would start over: one, two, pause."

Tests revealed Kay was experiencing what a lot of people describe as "skipped beats." In fact, these premature ventricular contractions are extra, abnormal heartbeats that begin in one of the heart's two ventricles. While many people have them throughout their lifetimes, and athletes even more so, Kay's heart was under huge stress, enduring upward of 30,000 PVCs per day. When you consider that an athlete will have about 80,000 heartbeats each day, Kay's heart was out of rhythm more than a third of the time.

Bigeminy (a PVC every other beat) and trigeminy (a PVC every third beat) lead to a chaotic heart with lower overall cardiac output. These uncoordinated contractions don't move blood very well; it's like going from a robust V8 to a sputtering four-cylinder engine. Sometimes the ventricle contracts against a closed valve. Sometimes it contracts and pushes a little blood, but the chamber isn't ready for it. After each PVC, the heart needs to pause and reset.

Kay's electrophysiologist first had him try conservative methods to alleviate the symptoms, things like yoga and meditation. Kay attempted to reduce stress in his life. He cut out coffee.

He did this for two months, but nothing changed. Further tests revealed there were no structural abnormalities, no obvious defects in the shape of the heart or clogged arteries. An ablation—a procedure to scar small areas of the heart to prevent the propagation of abnormal electrical signals (see Chapter 8)— was the next course of action.

During consecutive weeks, Kay spent more than 14 hours on the operating table. During the first ablation procedure, doctors were unable to find the exact location of the erratic cells. "The procedure is very inexact," Kay says. "It's kind of like pin the tail on the donkey. For hour after hour the technician is saying, 'Okay, move one millimeter to the left, move one millimeter up or down.' It's just hour after hour—'Is this it, is this it?' Then they cook it up; they probably burned 15 or 20 spots in my heart, but they never found the source—they never got it to stop."

The next week, the second ablation worked. A week later, Kay underwent a cardiac stress test on a treadmill; he was able to hit his maximum heart rate of 182 beats per minute and hasn't had any significant PVCs since.

Kay still exercises regularly, but he's decided that his racing career is over. "It's actually quite relieving," he says. "I've been racing since high school, first alpine, then racing endurance ski events since 1979." Nowadays, he says, he wakes up and thinks, "It's Sunday morning? Oh, I don't have to do a long workout; I can sit here and drink coffee! I'm okay with it; I've done enough racing."

Did his life of endurance training have anything to do with his arrhythmia? Kay is convinced it did. "I read all this stuff, and I think it's got to be related to this chronic inflammatory process," he says. "I was starting my own business in 2009, and you look at the stress load: the job stress, the life stress, the work stress, the training stress."

Because exercise is medicine, there's a dose response. Kay willingly admits he overdosed on it, and it led to a negative response. He remembers his coaches lecturing him and other members of the US Ski Team in the 1980s: "You need to look at your whole training load," they said. "Do you have exams now; do you have something big going on in your life? If you do, you need to back off from your training."

"I violated that principle, and I got stung," he says.

After an initial battle with feelings of guilt, of having done this to himself, Kay has accepted that an athletic lifestyle is and always has been one of the greatest aspects of his life. It helped him escape from a troubled teenage life. As a coach, it's allowed him to give wiser advice to his athletes. "My experience is that most people, when they first get started on this performance training, do way too much. If I can save some other people from this problem, that will be a great success," he says.

2 | The athlete's heart

LENNARD ZINN

IT SHOULD BE OBVIOUS that an athlete, by demanding more performance from his or her arms, legs, and core muscles than the nonathlete, simultaneously demands more performance from his or her heart. But do some of these demands create long-term damage? Researchers are only beginning to find out. Before we delve into the research in later chapters, let's first take a look at what the athlete asks of the heart that the nonathlete does not.

Number of total beats

The average adult male heart beats 72 times a minute at rest.[1] The average resting heart rate for females is 80 beats per minute. (A child's resting pulse might range from 90 to 120 beats per minute.) Assuming the same average rate while both sleeping and awake, this totals about 100,000 beats per day for men and 115,000 for women, about 38 million beats per year for men and 42 million for women, and about 3 billion beats during an 80-year lifetime for men and 3.4 billion for women.

Due to conditioning, an endurance athlete's heart tends to beat considerably slower than 72 bpm while at rest. The amount of blood the heart pumps in a given time period (cardiac output in liters per minute) is proportional to the size of the heart's stroke volume as well as to the heart rate. Due to the cardiac hypertrophy that is one component of a collection of features of cardiac adaptation to long-term exercise, a condition dubbed "Athlete's Heart," the left ventricle (the one that pumps blood throughout the body) becomes enlarged, allowing the heart to maintain sufficient blood flow to the body while beating at a lower rate (Figure 2.1). This is one of the reasons why athletes generally have lower resting heart rates than nonathletes.[2]

An athlete's heart also tends to get revved up to very high rates almost every day, often for many hours at a time. If the athlete's heart beats at 40 beats per minute during 8 hours of sleep per day, averages 60 bpm during waking hours, and then zooms up to 125 bpm for 3 hours of working out daily, then the daily total is actually less than the example above: around 88,000 beats per day, or 32 million beats per year and 2.5 billion beats during an 80-year lifetime. Three hours of aerobic exercise every day is already high for most athletes, but even if the athlete were to spend 6 hours per day working out at 125 bpm, assuming 40 bpm while sleeping for 8 hours and 60 bpm the rest of the time, the athlete's heart still beats fewer total beats in 80 years than if it had been averaging 72 bpm that entire time.

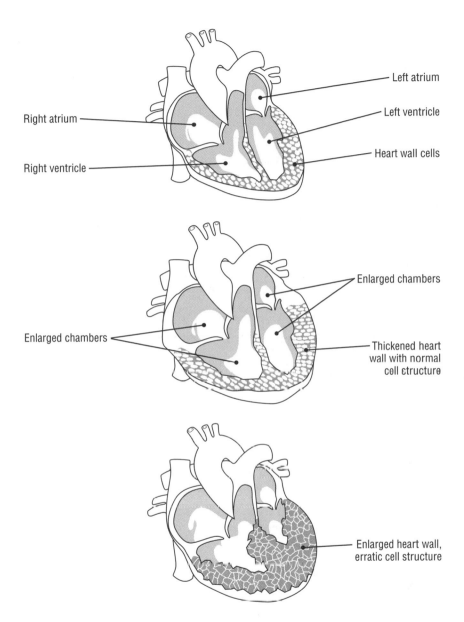

Left atrium

Left ventricle

Right atrium

Heart wall cells

Right ventricle

Enlarged chambers

Enlarged chambers

Thickened heart
wall with normal
cell structure

Enlarged heart wall,
erratic cell structure

FIGURE 2.1. Structural differences in the normal heart (top), the athlete's heart (middle), and a diseased heart suffering from hypertrophic cardiomyopathy (bottom)

Certainly during intense workouts, heart rates generally go much higher than 125 bpm, but this is counterbalanced by the fact that the higher the heart rate, the shorter the time it can be maintained. An average of 125 bpm over long endurance workouts as well as interval workouts with rest periods between is certainly in the ballpark. No matter how you slice it, it's likely the calculation for athletes will not yield significantly higher totals over 80 years than 3 billion beats for males and 3.4 billion beats for females.

Volume of blood pumped

At rest, the average male heart ejects around 70 ml (0.018 gallons) of blood with each contraction. At an average resting heart rate of 72 bpm, that is 1.3 gallons per minute. Since women are generally smaller than men and thus have smaller hearts, the ejection volume is lower, and hence the average resting heart rate may be higher. Since a man has an average of 5 liters (1.32 gallons) of total blood (women average 4 liters, or 1.06 gallons), this means that, at rest, the body circulates its entire volume of blood every minute.

At 200 bpm and 0.018 gallons per beat during intense exercise, this becomes 3.6 gallons per minute. In other words, the entire volume of blood in the body will be circulated nearly three times per minute when you are working out at your maximum rate. Taking into account the enlarged heart size that results from long-term training, it is estimated that some athletes pump up to 8 gallons of blood (30 liters, or six times the total blood volume of the average man) per minute during intense exercise.[3] A normal male heart weighs around 10.5 ounces (300 grams), whereas the average female heart is 9 ounces (250 grams). However, the hypertrophy of an athlete's heart can bring its weight up to 500 grams or more, which explains the higher volume of blood it can move through the body.

Imagine how much blood 8 gallons (or even 3.6 gallons) is; a kitchen faucet can take two minutes just to fill a 3-gallon bucket. Even while the body is resting, the heart is pumping almost as much blood as a kitchen faucet at full blast. And, let's not forget, blood is thicker than water. That is an awesome little pump we have in our chest.

Using that average blood output number of 1.3 gallons per minute, the average human heart pumps 78 gallons per hour, 1,872 gallons per day, or 683,280 gallons per year. Given that a railroad tank car holds about 30,000 gallons, the heart is filling the equivalent of 23 tank cars per year. In an 80-year lifespan, that's 55 million gallons of blood, enough to fill 1,833 railroad tank cars. To gush out the same amount of water as the blood a human heart pumps in an average lifetime, a kitchen faucet that flows 1.5 gallons per minute would need to be turned on full for over 69 years.

There are about 60,000 miles of blood vessels in the adult body, enough to wrap the earth's circumference twice with some left over (the earth's equator is only 25,000 miles around). Those vessels range in size from the aorta, which is nearly the diameter of a garden hose, to capillaries so thin that ten of them together are only as thick as a human hair.

The output of the heart is remarkable; so too is its endurance. Until your heart weakens for other reasons, it won't fatigue from pumping these massive volumes of blood day in and day out. Squeezing a tennis ball in your hand is similar to the force of a beating heart, yet there's no way you could do it 100,000 times a day as your heart does. And another 100,000 times tomorrow. And the day after that. And . . .

Blood pressure in athletes

In addition to a low resting heart rate, endurance athletes also tend to have low resting blood pressure. Their systolic pressure (the top number that represents the pressure when the heart muscle contracts) goes up less with exercise than it does in nonathletes. The increase in systolic blood pressure is generally under 50 percent and temporary. Diastolic blood pressure (when the heart relaxes) stays steady and may even drop during exercise due to blood-vessel dilatation.[4] These relaxation properties of exercise are important, in that they are probably one of the key ways by which regular exercise delivers health benefits.

Since it is the left ventricle that sends blood throughout the body, research on the work done by the right ventricle, which sends deoxygenated blood to the lungs, has lagged. However, it is often the one in which ventricular arrhythmias in athletes appear. The study of pulmonary artery hypertension (PAH) inevitably has led to investigation of the right ventricle, which is the pump that generates pulmonary pressure. To help understand how patients with PAH respond to submaximal exercise, studies have been performed on normal volunteers as well as on athletes.

The major differences between the left ventricular/arterial interaction and the right ventricular/pulmonary vascular system interaction can be found in the relative sizes of the two systems and their relative blood pressures. The total surface area of the body's arterial system is 800 to 1,000 square meters, compared with a surface area of only 80 to 100 square meters in the pulmonary vessels.[5] And while the blood pressure in arteries throughout the body is on the order of 120/70 mmHg in healthy people, blood pressure in the pulmonary vessels generally averages 20/8 mmHg.[6] The same amount of blood flows through the pulmonary system, yet the pressure in it at rest is only 10 to 20 percent as high.

The right ventricle in a trained athlete, however, has the power to greatly increase pressure in the pulmonary vascular system to maximize oxygen exchange in the lungs. Elite endurance athletes can see a more than fourfold increase in peak pulmonary pressures (pushed by the right ventricle) during exercise, while peak arterial systolic pressures (pushed by the left ventricle) may remain within 10 mmHg of the at-rest recordings.[7]

Increases in pulmonary blood pressure and corresponding increases in blood pressure in the right ventricle and left atrium (where the oxygenated blood from the lungs circulates to) may be variables that contribute to cardiac electrical problems in long-term elite athletes. Right ventricular and left atrial remodeling observed in these athletes can lead to the establishment of the compromised substrate required for arrhythmias to develop.[8] This will be discussed further in Chapter 4.

Heart power output

To compute the power output of the heart, we can multiply the blood pressure times the volume of blood flowing through the body per unit time.

To work in round numbers, consider a large person with 6 liters of blood. At resting heart rate, a person's entire blood volume circulates approximately once per minute, so the flow rate is 6 liters in 60 seconds, or 6,000 cm³ in 60 seconds = 100 cm³/s.

Again, to work in round numbers, consider the blood pressure to be 120/80 mmHg, so the average pressure (ignoring pulsations in flow) is

$$100 \text{ mmHg} = 10 \text{ cmHg} = 10 \times 1.33 \times 10^4 \text{ dynes/cm}^2 =$$
$$133{,}000 \text{ dynes/cm}^2.$$

The average power output is the pressure times the flow rate, or

$$133{,}000 \text{ dynes/cm}^2 \times 100 \text{ cm}^3/\text{s} = 1.33 \times 10^7 \text{ ergs/s} \times 10^{-7} \text{ joules/erg} =$$
$$1.33 \text{ J/s} = 1.33 \text{ watts}.$$

And when a highly trained athlete is circulating those 6 liters of blood three times per minute, rather than just once a minute, then the heart's power output jumps to

$$3 \times 1.33 \text{ W} = 4 \text{ watts}.$$

And in athletes who can move 8 gallons of blood per minute (30 liters), this becomes

$$5 \times 1.33 \text{ W} = 6.7 \text{ watts}.$$

When compared to a 100-watt lightbulb or the 400 watts you can get to appear on your bicycle power meter by pedaling hard, 1.33 W or even 4 W or 7 W may not seem like much. However, unlike the lightbulb or your legs, the heart continuously produces power for your entire lifetime. The amount of work done by the heart (its energy output) at rest in a day is

$$1.33 \text{ J/s} \times 24 \text{ hrs/day} \times 60 \text{ min/hr} \times 60 \text{ s/min} \sim 115{,}000 \text{ J/day}.$$

Compare this amount to the kinetic energy (KE) of a 100-kg (220-pound) boulder falling off a building. KE = mgh (m = mass in kilograms, g = acceleration due to gravity, and h = height in meters), so the height of the building, h, equals

$$h = KE/mg = 115{,}000 \text{ J} / 100\text{kg} / 9.8\text{m/s}^2 = 117\text{m} = 383 \text{ feet}.$$

So the heart produces as much energy in a single day as a 100-kg boulder does while falling from a building 383 feet tall (or as much energy as it would take to lift that boulder up to that height). That would leave a big dent in the sidewalk; 15 states in America don't even have a building tall enough to do this experiment!

The mechanical efficiency of the heart is less than 10 percent,[9] so the heart will demand over 10 times as much energy (in Calories) as it produces, or in this case, 10 × 115,000 J = 1,150,000 joules in a day, or

$$1.15 \times 10^6 \text{ J} \times 0.239 \text{ cal/J} \times 10^{-3} \text{ Cal/cal} = 275 \text{ Calories}.$$

In other words, your resting heart requires about one Clif Bar per day in order to keep ticking.

So that I could have round numbers in the calculations above, I used 6 liters of blood in the body, but the average man has about 5 liters, and the average woman has perhaps 4 liters. Using 4.5 liters of blood to simplify the final calculation below, the power output of the average human heart at rest would be one watt (1 J/s), rather than 1.33 watts.

The amount of power the heart constantly generates inside you is nothing to scoff at; the average human heart at a resting output of one watt for 80 years does this much work:

$$1 \text{ J/s} \times 80 \text{ yrs} \times 365 \text{ days/yr} \times 24 \text{ hrs/day} \times 60 \text{ min/hr} \times 60 \text{ s/min} =$$
$$2.5 \text{ gigajoules (in other words, 2.5 billion joules).}$$

And if this average-sized human were to spend a tenth of each day (2.4 hours) exercising at an average cardiac power output of 3 watts, this total would become 3 gigajoules (3 billion joules) of work done by the heart in a lifetime. You will never ride your bike enough to rack up that kind of total energy output on your power meter.

The takeaway

While an endurance athlete's heart may not beat as many times per year as a sedentary person's, it can pump out six times as much blood as a kitchen faucet will put out at full flow. And when it's pumping that much blood during an intense workout, it may endure sustained pulmonary blood pressures four times greater than those of the sedentary person's heart. When the workout is over, the heart keeps producing as much energy every day as a 220-pound boulder would represent in kinetic energy after falling from a 38-story building. It should be no surprise that the heart muscle will grow in size to deal with the extraordinary demands an endurance athlete puts on it decade after decade.

CASE STUDY
Jenni Lutze: Premature ventricular complexes
Diagnosed at age 56

CHRIS CASE

JENNI LUTZE never considered herself to be an athlete, let alone an endurance athlete. She grew up in an isolated rural area of South Australia, and her childhood days were filled with tennis matches and netball. It was when she started college in Adelaide that she began running after feeling she'd become lethargic. She also rode her bike everywhere since she didn't have a car. For the next four years she rode her bike every day and developed an even deeper love for running.

During the 10 years she lived in Adelaide, she started playing many different sports: touch football, lacrosse, volleyball, and hockey, among others. And she continued to run nearly every day. During this time she also began to compete, annually running the City to Bay, a 12-kilometer (7.5-mile) fun run, posting sub-50-minute times on several occasions. She completed the Greenbelt Marathon at the age of 25 in a time of 2:58.

"I was really enjoying running at this stage of my life and I remember playing lacrosse and then going for a run afterward! I was addicted!" Lutze says.

After traveling for a year at age 27, she returned to a small rural town called Coonalpyn, about 100 miles outside Adelaide.

She took up running casually again to build some fitness. But when her first child arrived at age 31, she hardly ran at all for the next decade.

By 2008, Lutze was back to competition, participating in a few local triathlons before joining a club in Adelaide in 2011. "This is what really gave me a taste for getting fit and participating in so many exciting events that happen around the country," she says. She gradually built up to the Olympic distance, competing in about 10 events during 2013 and 2014, winning many of them for her age group. She then completed a half-Ironman in Auckland in 2015.

When she turned 50, she decided she wanted to run a marathon. The first year into her plan she managed a half-marathon, building to a full marathon the next year. She ran it in 3:49, good enough to qualify for the New York City marathon. She set her mind to developing some good fitness.

Unfortunately, she missed her chance to compete in New York when Hurricane Sandy hit. Instead, she entered the first marathon she could back in Australia, the Gold Coast marathon. On a warm day, she ran it in 3:30. Her performance helped her get invited to compete in the Melbourne marathon as an elite. She couldn't turn down the offer.

With 14 weeks between the two events, Lutze volunteered for a research project that was investigating a training program involving two easy weeks, four hard weeks, and another two easy weeks. It was during this regimen that she first noticed her heart rate rising very high. The researchers said it was probably the heart rate monitor acting up.

Though she remembers having spikes in her heart rate as far back as 2012, twice in half-marathons, it would usually drop down if she backed off. But in October 2015, during the Australian Masters Games, that wasn't the case. Lutze was competing in the half-marathon as a 55-year-old. She got extremely lightheaded while pushing up a small incline and felt "really, really awful." She stopped to walk, felt worse, started running again, felt slightly better, and finished the race. Her heart rate was high by then, and it wouldn't subside even though she had slowed down. Her race time was 1:45, which was her slowest half-marathon in many years.

When she recently sifted through her archive of heart rate data, she found many races in which her heart rate exceeded 190 beats per minute. Normally, she says, it didn't bother her.

It was around this time that she became involved in the research of Adrian Elliot, a PhD in the University of Adelaide School of Medicine's Centre for Heart Rhythm Disorders.

Throughout the course of the next year she underwent echocardiograms, stress tests, CT angiograms, MRIs, blood tests, ECGs, and Holter monitoring. All these procedures revealed that the muscles, valves, and blood vessels of her heart were in very good order. It was the electrical system that wasn't functioning well. Elliot found that Lutze was having a relatively high number of premature ventricular complexes, about 17,000 per day, originating in the right ventricle. Her team of physicians recommended she have an ablation, but she'd have to wait seven months for that time to come.

"On echo and MRI, left ventricle and right ventricle structure and function are within normal limits," Elliot says. "There is mild atrial dilation consistent with that seen in athletes with similar training history. There is no evidence of infiltrative cardiomyopathy. Using a fairly crude questionnaire, I have estimated that her lifetime endurance training exceeds 6,000 hours."

Meanwhile, she was told to not let her heart rate rise above 180 beats per minute. She ran a few half-marathons in which she had to slow down to keep her heart rate below that threshold.

"Both times I ran a time of 1:42, which hurts when you get used to running 1:35 and are training to run faster and not slower!" Lutze says. Her next big races were at the Australian Athletics Masters Games in April 2016. She entered the 1,500-meter run and the 5K and the 8K cross-country events. She won silver and two golds. And she did it all while keeping her heart rate even lower. By now she had been told that 160 was to be her max.

She finally underwent the ablation procedure in June 2016. Two weeks after her symptoms were relieved, the palpitations returned.

What's worse, though, was that after another round of Holter monitoring and an MRI, she was found to be experiencing short episodes of what Elliot calls "complete heart block." The impulses generated from the heart's pacemaker (the SA node in the right atrium) weren't transmitting to the ventricles as they should. Consequently, there was complete disassociation between the electrical activity in the atria and ventricles. (In a healthy heart, they are tightly coordinated.) In Lutze's case, the contraction of the ventricles was instead being initiated by what is called an "escape" rhythm, which is generated from somewhere within the ventricles. It typically operates at a much lower rate, thus resulting in an abnormally low heart rate. Lutze was fitted with a pacemaker in August 2016.

"Now that I know it's not normal to get lightheaded often, I am very aware of it," she says. "With the pacemaker my heart rate will no longer drop below 50, which it often did for the past 15 years or so."

Weeks after the procedure, she was back to easy training and spin classes. "It does something for the soul to get out and run amongst the bush again," she says. She'll miss the City to Bay 12K this year for the first time in six years. "I don't like the idea of running an event where you pay an entry fee and just run casually. If I'm going to enter a race, I want to push myself to my limits. Yes, I have white-line fever."

She's not sure what she'll do next. Her cardiologist has said she should do nothing more than an hour of exercise at a time—no more marathons or triathlons. "My entire social life is based around being active," she says. "Right now I feel like I have a big hole left in my life and I'm just sitting around getting fat! I might have said goodbye to racing days."

So, after all these years of training and racing, does Lutze think endurance exercise contributed? She doesn't think so. She reasons that her father had a low heart rate, and there has been a history of heart disease in her family, hence her obsession with keeping fit. She has three sisters with hypothyroidism; her mother had it as well. (She also had CREST syndrome, or scleroderma.) She is still grappling with the idea of how this could have happened to her.

"Running has always been my path to good health," she says. "It has been a shock to be told that maybe it has contributed to my heart problems."

3 | Heart attacks, arrhythmias, and endurance athletes

JOHN MANDROLA

IN THE 1970S, James Fixx was an overweight, overstressed smoker with a precarious family history: His father had suffered a heart attack at the age of 35 and died eight years later from another. Rehabilitation of a tennis injury motivated Fixx to start running regularly. It eventually became his passion. His 1977 best selling book *The Complete Book of Running* is often credited with igniting America's fitness revolution, popularizing the sport of running, and demonstrating the health benefits of regular exercise.

That same year, Dr. Tom Bassler boldly theorized that the stress of running marathons built immunity to the development of fatty deposits within coronary arteries—that is, that running actually prevented coronary artery disease. Bassler compared marathon runners to the heart disease–free Masai warriors of East Africa and the Tarahumara Indians of northwestern Mexico in that they all maintained active lifestyles, ate healthful foods, and had enlarged and wide-bore coronary arteries.

Fixx's positive family history for heart disease and his love of running inclined him to agree with Bassler. Some have suggested that may be why Fixx ignored chest pains while he ran, hoping they would go away if he kept on running.

Unfortunately, his passion for running came to an end along a Vermont road in 1984 when, in the middle of a run at the age of 52, Fixx died of a heart attack. An autopsy found a complete blockage in one coronary artery, an 80 percent blockage in another, and signs of previous heart attacks.

In 1985, exercise physiologist Kenneth Cooper published *Running Without Fear: How to Reduce the Risk of Heart Attack and Sudden Death During Aerobic Exercise*. In it, he detailed the risk factors that might have contributed to Fixx's death. After reviewing Fixx's medical records and autopsy, and interviewing Fixx's friends and family, Cooper concluded that Fixx was genetically predisposed. In addition to his father's death from a heart attack, Fixx himself had a congenitally enlarged heart. Of course, his life before taking up running at age 36 was an unhealthy one. Fixx was a heavy smoker, had a stressful occupation, had suffered through two divorces, and had trouble controlling his weight, which had ballooned to 214 pounds.

Fixx's story helps emphasize an important point about exercise: While it can be protective, it is not a panacea. Neither running nor any other type of physical activity can undo years of neglect. Getting the exercise bug after decades of unhealthy living is surely a good thing, but it may not be able to undo the silent buildup of disease, and may play a role in some of the diseases observed in older endurance athletes.

Fixx's story also helps illustrate a few key points: First, not all "heart attacks" are created equal, as you'll learn in this chapter. Second, while heart attacks can strike athletes, too much exercise does not tend to cause them. (The same cannot be said about arrhythmias, which is why they are the main focus of this book.) Third, before we delve into the science of heart problems, we need to define the terminology you'll see throughout this book. Finally, it will be helpful to have an understanding of the heart conditions we are *not* talking about in this book.

Heart attack (myocardial infarction)

Let's begin this discussion of common heart problems with an often misunderstood term: heart attack. The phrase itself can be confusing because it is regularly, if incorrectly, applied to all manner of heart troubles. The more precise medical term for a heart attack is "myocardial infarction" (MI). The myocardium is the middle, muscular layer of the heart wall, and "infarction" refers to the death of an area of the muscle due to an abrupt blockage of a blood vessel that supplies blood to it. A heart attack, therefore, is a problem with the "plumbing" of the heart itself rather than disruption of the electrical impulses that set the heart's rhythm. (Jim Fixx had an MI.) The blood vessels that nourish the heart are called the coronary arteries, and they lie on the outside of the heart. Like any blood vessel in the body, they are susceptible to blockages.

The coronary arteries arise from the aorta, the main vessel coming out of the heart. During the relaxation phase between heartbeats, blood flows down the coronary arteries to the contracting heart. (The heart's chambers, which we'll soon describe in more detail, may be filled with blood, but that blood inside the heart does the beating muscle no good. Just like a bicep or thigh muscle, the heart muscle needs its own blood supply.)

When drawn on paper, coronary arteries look like simple pipes, but in reality the walls of these arteries, called endothelia, are teeming with activity. Endothelial cells grow, secrete chemical messengers, slough off, and sometimes break. Meanwhile, platelets, the "sticky" cells in blood involved in clotting, interact physically and chemically with these active endothelial cells in the arterial wall.

In the typical form of heart disease, problems arise in the interaction of blood and the arterial wall. If the endothelium becomes inflamed, it is more apt to swell (with fatty deposits), more apt to redden (with blood clots), and more apt to scar. This hardening of the arteries is called atherosclerosis.

Because this is a book about endurance exercise and heart disease, the concept of inflammation deserves a brief explanation. Inflammation is a normal process by which the body repairs and protects itself from harmful stimuli. Inflammation is essential for life. When you are infected with a virus or injured in a bike crash, for example, the inflammatory response clears the virus or repairs the injured tissue. Fever caused by an infection or muscle soreness caused by a hard workout are due to inflammation. These are examples of acute inflammation. Sustained irritation of the body can cause prolonged or chronic inflammation. Smoking is a common cause of chronic inflammation. Continued exposure to tobacco leads to inflammation of the inside of the arteries. Other diseases of the immune system, such as lupus and rheumatoid arthritis, link to chronic inflammation.

Inflammation also activates platelets, making them stickier and therefore more likely to clot and attach to the inflamed endothelium. A blood clot that attaches to an inflamed blood vessel wall is the most common cause of heart attacks. This is true for women and men alike.

When a supplying vessel becomes obstructed, the part of the heart downstream is injured. If the blockage is not opened, the local muscle tissue infarcts, or dies.

Injury of the heart is often felt as chest pain, tightness, or breathlessness. In the same way that a too-tight tourniquet on an arm will cause the hand to hurt, the injured heart usually produces discomfort (though one in ten heart attacks can be silent). If injury continues for more than a few minutes, death of the muscle creates scar tissue, which is permanent. The symptoms of lack of blood to the heart (or ischemia) vary considerably. Sometimes a small area of heart damage will cause a lot of pain in one patient, while a massive heart attack causes little to no pain in another. Doctors don't understand why people feel heart symptoms so differently.

Until recently, there was no way to stop a heart attack. Nowadays, however, abrupt blockages of coronary arteries can be opened either with a clot-busting drug or, more commonly, with an angioplasty procedure that squishes the blockage against the artery walls at the site, after which the area is propped open with a metal mesh tube called a stent.

Not all heart attacks are fatal, and while heart attacks can and do happen to athletes, we should emphasize again that exercise alone—even in the high doses commonly pursued by endurance athletes—does not tend to cause heart attacks. When they strike lifelong athletes, however, they seem to take on an air of mystery. How could this happen to someone so fit?

You may recall the story of Cuban-born track coach and former world-class long-distance runner Alberto Salazar, who is best known for his performances in the New York City Marathon in the early 1980s (when he won three consecutive editions) and his race with Dick Beardsley in the 1982 Boston Marathon, known as the "Duel in the Sun." More recently, he gained attention for being felled by a heart attack on June 30, 2007, that nearly killed him. He was only 48 years old, and the news caused convulsions throughout the running community.

Unlike Fixx, Salazar survived his heart attack. But their stories had many similarities. In an effort to educate other runners about the risk of heart attack, Salazar allowed his cardiologist to speak to *Runner's World* about his case. Dr. Todd Caulfield, MD, the medical director for interventional cardiology research at Provident St. Vincent Medical Center in Portland, Oregon, first met Salazar on the morning of the athlete's heart attack.

He reported that Salazar had a number of risk factors: a family history of coronary disease, high blood pressure, and high cholesterol, the latter two of which were being controlled with medications. His being male was a risk factor, too, since males have a higher statistical incidence of MI than females. "Even when you control for heart-disease risk factors, they still persist as risk factors. You can't completely mitigate against them," Dr. Caulfield said.

Arrhythmia

Unlike an MI, which affects the heart muscle, an arrhythmia, or abnormal rhythm, is a problem with the electrical system of the heart. That electrical system comprises two parts: special cells embedded within the heart's muscle, and the heart muscle cells themselves.

As discussed in Chapter 1, the sinoatrial (SA) node and atrioventricular (AV) node have similar specialized properties. First, the SA node generates the heartbeat, and then the AV node and His-Purkinje bundles transmit it. (The AV node can sometimes have heartbeat-generating properties.) These cells can be seen under a microscope; they look different than regular muscle fibers. Some people call them the specialized conduction system.

The role of the heart muscle cells is to transmit the electrical signal throughout the chambers from cell to cell; this signal rolls through the heart in a wave of sorts. When the special cells and muscle cells conduct electricity properly, the heart's rhythm is smooth and regular. This wave idea is key to understanding the heart rhythm. Problems with cell-to-cell transmission of the electrical impulses give rise to many sorts of arrhythmias.

You may wonder what the difference is between the special cells and heart muscle cells. It's a good question. For one, there are some chemical differences (mainly the SA node and AV node conduct more slowly). For the purposes of understanding rhythm problems, the key is thinking about a smooth wave of conduction. Things that disrupt smooth wave-like conduction of electricity can affect special cells and muscle cells.

Arrhythmia, then, is any abnormality of electrical impulse generation or conduction through the heart. There are many reasons why this wave of electricity could be disrupted. We will talk more about specific types of rhythm problems later, but let's start with the scariest.

Ventricular fibrillation

The most malignant form of arrhythmia is sudden cardiac death (SCD) due to ventricular fibrillation (VF). This is called cardiac arrest.

Fibrillation is a medical term referring to a superfast heart rate—greater than 300 beats per minute. At that rate, the heart cannot fill properly with blood. Consequently, little to no blood is pumped from the heart to the body. Without blood, the organs, especially the brain, stop working, usually within seconds of the VF event.

Electrically, the problem is that the heart is going so fast it can't squeeze blood. Therefore, the word "arrest" in the phrase "cardiac arrest" pertains to the mechanical standstill of the heart's ability to pump blood.

But here is the confusing part: An abrupt closure of an artery—a heart attack—is a common cause of VF and, therefore, cardiac arrest and sudden death. In this case, the disruption of cell-to-cell transmission of impulses induces VF and cardiac arrest. We will keep coming back to that mechanism, because it bears on nearly all the heart's rhythm problems.

When an athlete dies suddenly, either during competition or at rest, determining whether it was due to a heart attack (blockage) or sole electrical event (ventricular fibrillation) turns on age. Most experts use 35 years as the cutoff. In reality, the dividing line is a bit arbitrary. In most athletes under 35 who die suddenly, the VF event is not caused by a blockage. In athletes over 35 years of age, the cause of sudden death is usually an electrical problem caused by a blockage.

The good news is that fibrillation of the pumping chambers, either due to a blockage or electrical event, is rare.

Additional heart problems

Most of this book focuses on the rhythm problems of the heart that strike athletes and the growing evidence that links intense exercise to arrhythmia (that evidence is the subject of the next chapter). Before we move on to common rhythm problems, though, it's worth touching on other causes of cardiac arrest or sudden death.

Hypertrophic cardiomyopathy

We will look at this topic further in a later chapter, but in short, hypertrophic cardiomyopathy (HCM) is an abnormal thickening of the heart's muscle that is usually concentrated in the septum between the left and right ventricles. It usually afflicts athletes younger than 35 and is usually caused by abnormal genes, which means that it is generally a disease one is born with, although it may not become apparent until the late teens or early 20s.

Cardiomyopathy

Cardiomyopathy is a medical term for any heart muscle disease. These diseases can range from conditions someone is born with (familial cardiomyopathy), to acquired cardiomyopathy (caused by a virus or alcohol abuse) and even an acute infection (myocarditis).

Two interesting forms of cardiomyopathy we discuss later are arrhythmogenic right ventricular cardiomyopathy (ARVC) and Phidippides cardiomyopathy. They deserve our attention because they may be acquired or modified by endurance exercise.

Long QT syndrome and other inherited abnormalities of heart ion channels

The most common form of disease that affects the heart ion channels is Long QT syndrome. As we discussed in Chapter 1, "ion" is a term for atoms or molecules that carry a net electrical charge, either positive or negative. In the heart the most important ions are sodium, potassium, and calcium. These elements traverse the heart's cell membranes with every contraction. Proteins group together in the cell membrane to form channels. People can inherit abnormal genes that control these proteins, and the abnormality can lead to disrupted electrical conduction through the heart. Long QT syndrome mostly affects young, often very young, athletes. And fortunately, it's rare.

Pulmonary embolism

A blood clot in a pulmonary artery or one of its branches is called a pulmonary embolism (PE), and just one of these clots can cause sudden cardiac arrest. A PE occurs when a clot forms in the veins, often in the pelvis or legs, and then breaks free to travel through the veins to the heart, where it is then pumped toward the lungs through the pulmonary arteries. Three conditions, summed up in Virchow's Triad (named after Dr. Rudolf Virchow, a 19th-century German doctor) favor the formation of these blood clots in the veins: stasis, trauma, and hypercoaguable state.

The body's overall physical movement helps blood move through veins. (It's why doctors get patients up and out of bed as soon as possible after surgery.) An injury of or near a vein, say from surgery or a bike crash, sets off the body's clotting system. That's what is supposed to happen, but in the presence of poor blood movement (sitting through an 8-hour car ride after a faraway bike race, for example) these clots can enlarge and then move northward to the lungs.

A hypercoaguable state refers to a condition in which the blood is more apt to clot than normal. Infection, inflammatory processes, and cancer are conditions that can cause hypercoaguable states. Uncommonly, people can harbor a higher tendency of clotting from birth.

When clots in the veins travel to the lungs, they cause the heart to fail due to pressure overload and low oxygen levels (because the clot blocks blood from getting oxygenated in the lungs). The good news for athletes is that pulmonary embolism is uncommon, and sudden death from it is rare. (Although clots in the veins are rare, they are not unheard-of in athletes who endure long periods of travel after major events.)

Aortic tear

Another rare cause of cardiac arrest in athletes is a tear in the aorta, the main blood vessel coming out of the heart. The medical term for this problem is "aortic dissection," and it's often due to an inherited condition in which the lining of the blood vessel is weaker than normal. Abnormal valves can also cause problems with the aorta, which is sort of good news, because valve problems can be detected on an exam (doctors hear a heart murmur). Among athletes, cases of abrupt tears of the aorta are most often described in resistance-sports participants, such as weight lifters.

All this talk of heart attacks, cardiac arrest, and blood clots sounds terrible. The good news for athletes is that many of them are unlikely to strike healthy, active people, and most rhythm problems are not deadly.

Nonlethal arrhythmias—from either the atrium or ventricle—may be serious: They may lead to loss of consciousness, they may have an impact on lifestyle, and they may require treatment. But most do not lead to death without warning. It's worth repeating that sentence: The great majority of heart rhythm problems are not lethal!

You may ask, then, why begin a discussion with the least common and most deadly rhythm problems?

Well, that is how the practice of medicine works. A doctor's first concern is the risk of death. When a patient voices complaints that could be due to a heart problem, doctors first decide the potential for death. We call this initial sorting-out process "risk stratification." Basically, we decide the pace of the evaluation.

The way doctors approach this initial sorting-out process is to determine the company the arrhythmia or arrhythmia-symptoms keep. Consider these two examples:

Case 1. An accomplished 16-year-old cross-country runner faints on the starting line of a big race. She has, for years, passed all of her pre-participation exams; she has no medical problems, takes no medications, has no family history of heart disease. But she does have a history of fainting in stressful situations. That history alone suggests a benign cause of fainting, called vasovagal episodes. If her physical exam and basic ECG show no abnormality, she can be placed in a low-risk (not scary) category. Long may her running career continue.

Case 2. For comparison, consider a 65-year-old newcomer to triathlon who reports chest discomfort and a racing pulse during training. This man is 50 pounds overweight, quit smoking only months ago, and had a brother who died suddenly. Without even examining him, we are already worried about a high-risk (scary) plumbing or structural problem with his heart. We put this man in a much different risk category. Further tests should be conducted as soon as possible, and he should not train until this is sorted out.

Remember, the heart's electrical system is embedded within the heart's muscle. This means we must always consider the company a heart rhythm problem keeps.

What about atherosclerosis?

Most of this book deals with heart rhythm problems related to the endurance athlete. It would be easy to brush aside the run of the mill hardening of the arteries (atherosclerosis)—the disease that afflicts the overweight smoker who does not exercise. But we can't exclude standard atherosclerosis from our discussion.

The above case involving the 65-year-old newbie explains why this is so: Many of the athletes participating in today's boom in endurance sports are old enough to have atherosclerotic disease.

Remember, the cause of sudden cardiac death in competitive sports turns on age—under age 35, the cause is most often due to a born-with (inherited or congenital) problem, while over age 35, the cause is mostly due to blockage in a coronary artery. Since many endurance athletes are over 35, atherosclerosis cannot be excluded from the discussion.

Who's an athlete, who's a master, and what's an endurance sport?

The dictionary says an athlete is a person who is proficient in sports and other forms of physical exercise. In medical parlance, regular endurance exercise is defined as planned, structured, and repetitive movement for greater than 30 minutes at least three times per week for the purpose of increasing endurance. We would argue that an athlete is one who does at least this amount of exercise, usually much more, for many years in an attempt to compete. That competition doesn't have to be formal; we, and likely you, know plenty of people who exercise intensely over decades but rarely, if ever, pay an entry fee for a race. But the heart knows not whether it's in a sanctioned race or not. The heart knows only the dose of exercise.

When do athletes step over the threshold to become masters? That's a good question, and there's no firm answer. Most of the evidence discussed in this book deals with individuals older than 40, in part because age 40 is when the masters age-graded categories begin in most competitive endurance events. That seems like a reasonable cutoff, though we concede it's arbitrary.

As for what constitutes an endurance sport, let's simply say it is any prolonged muscle movement that requires high cardiac output. Examples include running, cycling, cross-country skiing, swimming, and triathlon.

We will spend little time in this book on resistance sports, such as weight lifting, American football, and sprint categories in track and field. These activities place different demands on the heart, and are rarely practiced for decades.

Exercise dosage

Hippocrates said, "The sick will of course profit to a great extent from gymnastics with regard to the restoration of their health, and the healthy will profit with regard to its maintenance, and those who exercise will profit with regard to the maintenance of their well-being and a lot more."

In other words, a lack of exercise is bad; regular amounts of exercise are good. Hundreds, perhaps thousands, of scientific citations support the benefits of regular, even vigorous exercise. Here are two studies that suggest "regular" exercise reduces the chance of getting the common heart rhythm condition called atrial fibrillation.

In terms of the heart rhythm, a study of older men and women whose histories were followed in four US communities for years found that those who walked the most had the lowest risk of developing atrial fibrillation.[1] Similarly, Dr. Peter Ofman and his colleagues from Harvard Medical School analyzed and combined four previous studies (called a meta-analysis) of more than 95,000 subjects and found no association between regular exercise and increased risk of atrial fibrillation.[2]

During the course of this book, we will discuss endurance athletes who develop heart rhythm problems. A question we will get close to answering but never be able to exactly quantify is, how much exercise is too much? What the judge said about pornography also applies to exercise dosage: We know it when we see it. You probably do too.

Can too much exercise kill you? As we mentioned at the beginning of this chapter, in the overwhelming majority of cases the answer is no. In other cases, the answer may very well be yes. And that's what we'll look at next.

CASE STUDY
Micah True: Undiagnosed

CHRIS CASE

Micah True went off alone on a Tuesday morning to run through the rugged trails of the Gila Wilderness in southwestern New Mexico. He was wearing only shorts, a T-shirt, and running shoes. It was late March 2012.

By Saturday, he hadn't returned. Rescue teams fanned out for 50 yards on each side of the marked trails, searching for any signs of the missing man. Riders on horseback crashed through the brush, past piñons, junipers, and ponderosa pines. An airplane and a helicopter circled above, zooming above the ridges and river canyons, looking for True.

True clearly had loyal friends. But he also had a devoted following, a product of the fame that had come by way of his depiction in Christopher McDougall's wildly popular 2009 book *Born to Run*—and because of his place as a legend in the sport of ultrarunning. Often called "Caballo Blanco" (Spanish for "white horse"), the 58-year-old was a mythic figure, known to compete in races two, three, and sometimes even four times as long as marathons. The day he disappeared, he said he was going on a 12-mile run. For True, that was just routine.

Born Michael Randall Hickman, True was often seen as a free spirit. Some say he survived on cornmeal and beans, shunning money and possessions. He spent several months per year during the 1980s and 1990s trail running in Central America. In 2003 he decided to organize a race for the Tarahumara people in Mexico that would help them preserve their culture and running heritage. Eventually, he called the remote Copper Canyons of northern Mexico home so he could be near the reclusive Tarahumara, believed to be the greatest natural runners in the world.

The volume of running True participated in, from training to racing to roaming, was legendary. He was reportedly logging about 170 miles a week in the late 1980s. The day before he died, he had gone for a six-hour run.

On March 27, 2012, True was found dead, lying face-up in a creek. The New York Times reported, "His body was reclining on an outcropping of small rocks and boulders. His legs were in 10 inches of water, and his arms were against his chest, the right one down, the left one up. One of his shoes was off, and nearby was a plastic water bottle, two-thirds empty."[3]

Were you one of the countless athletes—who likely started running or riding or exercising because you thought it was good for your health—who found the news shocking?

The most significant findings of True's autopsy were the presence of dilated cardiomyopathy and mild dehydration. His heart's left ventricle was reported to be "dilated and enlarged." Dilated cardiomyopathy is often idiopathic, meaning no cause can be identified. In this disease, the heart becomes enlarged due to dilation of the tissue, not due to increased thickness of the wall of the ventricle (as in left ventricular hypertrophy). The effect is a thin and enlarged heart wall that, like an overstretched water balloon, is too thin to contract effectively to pump blood to the rest of the body. The total volume of the heart is increased, but only because the wall of the heart has become thinner.

The autopsy also reported, "Microscopically there was no evidence of chronic ischemia, inflammation, or disarray of the myocardial architecture."

However, when Dr. James O'Keefe Jr., the director of the Preventive Cardiology Fellowship Program and the director of Preventive Cardiology at Cardiovascular Consultants at the Saint Luke's Mid America Heart Institute, looked at the autopsy report, he came to a slightly different conclusion. He believes that True's enlarged, thickened heart with scar tissue is a pathology that some extreme endurance athletes develop; it's termed "Phidippides cardiomyopathy." Justin E. Trivax and Peter A. McCullough conducted research that led to the hypothesis that "this pathology occurs because endurance sports call for a sustained increase in cardiac output for several hours," which puts the heart "into a state of volume overload. It has been shown that approximately one-third of marathon runners experience dilation of the right atrium and ventricle, have elevations of cardiac troponin and natriuretic peptides, and in a smaller fraction later develop small patches of cardiac fibrosis that are the likely substrate for ventricular tachyarrhythmias and sudden death."[4]

Unfortunately, the autopsy report can't tell us definitively what killed Micah True. The medical examiner who performed the autopsy deemed True's death a result of unclassified cardiomyopathy that resulted in a cardiac dysrhythmia during exertion. Alone in the woods, far from anyone, it became a medical emergency. There he died.

We will review the evidence at the core of this debate in the next chapter. For now, True's story serves as a reminder that even though, as someone who regularly exercises, you may feel completely healthy (perhaps even immortal), regular health screenings are essential. It is during these examinations that conditions like cardiomyopathy can be diagnosed.

4 | The evidence

JOHN MANDROLA

AS MENTIONED in the Introduction, the scientific research on high-dose exercise and its effects on the heart is difficult to tease out. It can often be more speculative than other types of medical research. In part that's because blinded randomized controlled trials, the strongest type of research method, are impossible to conduct in endurance athletes.

Yet a mountain of data exists, ranging from epidemiologic and observational studies to conclusions drawn from research in animals. Other findings drawn from looking at the heart muscle itself—for example, imaging studies that investigate changes in volume and scarring—also indicate there are connections and patterns not to be discounted.

In total, the evidence can't be ignored. Let's take a look.

Atrial fibrillation

The evidence supporting an association between atrial fibrillation and endurance exercise comes mostly from epidemiologic studies, which are observational studies of populations. Numerous animal and basic physiological (mechanistic) studies support the patterns seen in the observational studies. After reviewing these studies, we'll make the case that when taken together, excess endurance exercise could cause AF.

Before we describe the evidence, it's important to emphasize that this is more than a curious or academic matter. It's a critical argument because medical treatment works best when directed at the right target. Think of the treatment of infections. In a patient with muscle pain and fever from a bacterial infection, the correct treatment is not pain medications alone; it is antibiotics. That's because the real cause of the aches and fevers is the bacteria.

It is the same for AF. In the past, doctors considered AF its own disease. They put AF in a list of problems. A person could have diabetes, high blood pressure, and AF; three problems meant three different treatments. The new understanding of AF is more like that of fevers and aches from a bacterial infection. That is, AF is not a disease but a manifestation of other diseases acting on the atria.

It's long been known that high levels of thyroid hormone cause AF. When this occurs, fixing the thyroid usually resolves the AF. Likewise, patients with pericarditis, an inflammation of the lining of the heart, frequently develop AF. Once again, AF subsides once the inflammation is relieved. It's the same in patients with heart valve disease: Fix the valve and AF often resolves.

New thinking on AF extends these ideas. We now understand that common lifestyle problems lead to inflammation and atrial stretch. Obesity, sleep apnea, and high blood pressure, for instance, are three conditions strongly associated with AF.

Although the connection should have been obvious, many experts now believe excess inflammation and atrial stretch are the common links connecting lifestyle conditions with AF. The strongest evidence for this line of reasoning is that treatment of these risk factors reduces and often eliminates AF.[1] As in patients with thyroid and valve disease and pericarditis, removal of the stimulus for AF eliminates the AF.

If the atria fibrillate in response to inflammation and excess atrial stretch, it becomes easier to see how long-term intense endurance exercise might cause AF.

Epidemiologic or observational evidence

Numerous investigators have addressed the incidence of AF in athletes. The subjects in these various studies comprised orienteers, marathon runners, elite cyclists, and cross-country skiers. In 2009, Drs. Jawdat Abdulla and Jens Nielsen of Glostrup University in Copenhagen, Denmark, performed a meta-analysis of six case-controlled studies of 655 athletes and 895 control subjects.[2] They found AF in 23 percent of athletes and 12.5 percent of controls. Their conclusion was that being an endurance athlete increased one's odds of having AF fivefold. You can see a summary of these studies in Table 4.1.

More recently, a Scandinavian research team used data from the Birkebeiner Aging Study (BIAS), a longitudinal study of skiers aged 65 years and older participating in the Norwegian Birkebeiner cross-country ski race, to study the associations between long-term exercise and health in advanced age.[4]

At 54 kilometers in distance and with multiple climbs, the Birkebeiner cross-country ski race is among the world's most challenging. The research team compared 509 nonelite elderly men (65–90 years) who participated in the race with 1,768 men from the general population. Athletes were 1.9 times more likely to have AF than the controls. The finding is lower than in the Abdulla and Nielsen study. The Norwegian authors suggest this may be due to the higher percentage of AF in their control group. Remember, AF incidence increases with age, and this Norwegian study enrolled older subjects and older controls.

In 2013, Dr. Kasper Anderson and his Swedish colleagues studied more than 52,000 finishers of the Vasaloppet cross-country ski race over

Author/Year	Type of Athlete	Age (years)	Men %	Cases of AF/ Athletes	Cases of AF/ Controls
Karjalainen et al. 1998	Orienteers	42–54	100	12/28 (5%)	2/212 (0.9%)
Heidbüchel et al. 2006	Mixed sports	45–65	88	25/31 (81%)	50/106 (48%)
Elosua et al. 2006	Mixed sports	31–55	89	16/31 (51%)	35/129 (27%)
Molina et al. 2008	Marathoners	35–55	100	9/183 (5%)	2/290 (0.7%)
Mont et al. 2008	Mixed sports	38–58	100	83/120 (69%)	24/96 (25%)
Baldesberger et al. 2008	Cyclists	60–74	100	6/62 (10%)	0/62 (0%)
Total studies ($n = 6$)	Mixed sports	44–60	93	151/655 (23%)	113/895 (12.5%)

TABLE 4.1. Summary of Six Studies from Abdulla and Nielsen[3]

a 10-year period. They observed any type of arrhythmia in 919 athletes. Two factors increased the odds of AF: the number of times doing the race and a faster finishing time. Racers who completed five races were 29 percent more likely to have AF than those who completed only one. Athletes with the fastest finishing time were 30 percent more likely to have AF than those in the slowest group.[5]

Gender differences

You may have noticed that most of the studies mentioned thus far included mostly male athletes. In the nonathletic population, males are at greater risk for AF, although females with AF have a higher stroke risk. In 2011, Swiss researchers studied racers of the 10-mile running race called the Grand Prix of Bern to test the theory that male athletes were more prone to AF.[6] They randomly selected about 70 male and 70 female finishers. The two groups were well matched in age, lifetime training hours, and race time. Four male athletes (3.3 percent) and none of the female athletes developed AF during the follow-up period. The authors speculated that women's smaller atrial volume, lower blood pressure, and greater variability of heart rate protected them from AF.

Body stature

Men may be more susceptible to AF because of their larger stature. Larger people have larger hearts, and larger atria increase susceptibility to AF. In animal studies, AF is more common and more easily induced in larger species. A number of human studies support this finding.

Researchers at Emory University studied more than 7,000 patients with AF (whose average age was 66) who were enrolled in a registry for

patients with reduced heart pumping function.[7] The prevalence of AF
increased in taller subjects. The relationship between height and AF persisted after correcting for other factors. These patients did have heart
failure, however, so this study is less conclusive than the others.

Tall athletes

Spanish researchers reported a series of 107 patients (whose average age
was 48) who presented to the emergency department with new-onset
AF.[8] The research team split the group into three subgroups according
to height. Compared to patients with normal height, those in the tallest
group were 17 times more likely to have AF.

And German researchers compared 33 former top-level handball players (whose average age was 57) to age-matched controls.[9] Ten of the 33
athletes had AF. Athletes in the AF group were significantly taller than
those in the non-AF group.

Triggers and the atrial substrate

In all species, atrial fibrillation begins with triggers. The triggers are actually premature beats that most often occur from the left atrium (LA) in
the vicinity of the pulmonary veins (PV). The PV-LA junction is an important area for triggering of arrhythmia. It is beyond the scope of this book
to explain all the reasons for this, but one critical aspect of this junction,
especially relevant to athletes, is that this is the where the involuntary
nervous system connects to the heart.

We call these bundles of nerves "autonomic ganglia." The term "autonomic" refers to the involuntary nervous system, which controls things

like the heart. The sympathetic component of the autonomic nervous system works through adrenaline to raise the heart rate and blood pressure, while the parasympathetic component works through the vagus nerve and is responsible for low heart rates during periods of rest. When parasympathetic tone is high—during rest, after meals or training sessions, or during sleep—doctors say vagal tone is high.

A ganglia is a bundle of nerves. Stimulation of these ganglia in animal models can cause marked changes in the electrical properties of the heart, including induction of premature beats and AF.

But triggers are not the only requirement for AF. The atrial muscle itself is also vital for perpetuating AF. Doctors call the atrial muscle the "substrate." This substrate must be abnormal for AF to be sustained for any length of time. Typical conditions that cause an abnormal atrial substrate are inflammation, stretch, atria enlargement, and scarring.

When there is disease in the atria, triggers can induce and lead to sustained AF. An oversimplified way of thinking of sustained AF in diseased atria is to picture the rotation of a hurricane around its eye. You cannot get rotation of electrical impulses in atrial muscle unless there are patchy areas of substrate (from scar tissue, for example). A normal atrium only allows for normal conduction, and the premature beats cannot lead to sustained AF. Premature beats may be felt as an abnormal or irregular rhythm, but in the absence of an abnormal atrial substrate, they are usually extinguished without causing AF.

If the previously cited studies on populations are true, and endurance exercise does indeed promote AF, there should be biological plausibility.

And indeed, there are a number of studies we can look at that suggest endurance athletics might provide the means for both abnormal triggers and an abnormal substrate—and thus AF.

Triggers

In an elegant series of experiments using isolated canine heart muscle, a group of researchers from the University of Oklahoma (which has been and still is an epicenter for arrhythmia research) made the connection between stimulation of these autonomic ganglia and the triggering of premature beats that started AF.[10] They showed that triggered firing within the muscle sleeves of pulmonary veins required *combined* parasympathetic and sympathetic nerve stimulation. Yes, firing within veins required both parts of the involuntary nervous system.

The key finding of these experiments that relates to athletes is that repeated endurance exercise induces both intense sympathetic stimulation (during intense exercise) and profound parasympathetic predominance (due to the fitness accumulation). In other words, endurance athletes routinely experience both extremely high and extremely low heart rates. This back and forth may create the milieu that triggers premature beats, which could then induce AF.

Substrate

The most influential study on mechanisms of AF in athletes comes from the laboratory of Dr. Stanley Nattel at the Montreal Heart Institute and University of Montreal, in Quebec, Canada. His research group has previously shown that exercise training induced electrical and structural remodeling of the rat ventricle. (We will discuss the famous "marathon rat" study in the section on ventricular arrhythmias.) It may seem strange to use the word "beautiful" to describe an experiment, but any fan of biology would consider this truly beautiful work.

In the experiment, lead author Dr. Eduard Guasch and colleagues studied the effects of endurance exercise on the atria. They trained male rats to run one hour per day, five days per week, for up to 16 weeks. They chose this regimen because it simulated decades of training in a human. To be fair, other experts argued that the rats were overexercised.[11]

Compared with the sedentary control group, exercised rats showed evidence of enhanced vagal tone (lower heart rates), atrial dilation, atrial fibrosis (scarring), and enhanced vulnerability to AF. To test whether vagal stimulation was important for AF vulnerability, the investigators used the drug atropine, which blocks the effects of vagal stimulation on the heart. Indeed, atropine prevented vulnerability to AF. That was a key finding because it implied that low heart rates from high vagal tone are important for AF.

Detraining of the exercised rats resulted in rapid reversal of the vagal enhancement and AF vulnerability. Fibrosis and left atrial dilation, however, remained after the rats stopped exercising. (We will talk more about detraining in Chapter 8, which covers treatment options. Meanwhile, you may want to read this key paragraph again.)

The research team then explored the reasons for the enhanced vagal effects. They found that it was not just due to more outflow from the vagus nerve, but also, the exercised heart became more sensitive to the vagal stimulation. Researchers call this "enhanced end-organ sensitivity."

It's similar to when training makes your muscles more efficient at extracting nutrients.

Finally, the investigators looked for molecular reasons for enhanced vagal sensitivity of the exercised heart. Through a series of complex experiments, they found altered genetic expression of important intracellular signaling chemicals. That's right: Chronic exercise altered genetic components of the cells. The phenomenon by which external or environmental factors alter gene expression is called epigenetics.

These findings have major implications for the cardiac effects of endurance exercise. The experiment reproduced many of the findings of the athletic condition, such as lower heart rates and dilation of the atria. The exercised rats developed scarring in their atria. Scarring plus dilation plus greater sensitivity to vagal stimulation provides the abnormal substrate needed to maintain AF in athletes.

A second animal study

Replication is a key component of good science. An independent experiment that is able to corroborate previous findings serves to strengthen the initial conclusions. This is exactly what a different group of Canadian researchers did with the remarkable insights from Dr. Nattel's team, only with an extra twist. As was done with rats in the previous study, these researchers from Toronto exposed male mice to a six-week training regimen.[12] Compared to a group of sedentary mice, the trained group had lower heart rates, enlarged atria and ventricles, and atrial fibrosis (scarring). The trained mice in this study also had enhanced vulnerability to AF. This confirmed the findings of Guasch, Nattel, and colleagues.

The twist? The group also studied the possible role of inflammation in causing the fibrosis and enhanced vulnerability to AF. They considered an odd-sounding cell-signaling protein called "tumor necrosis factor" (TNF). The research team felt that TNF was a viable candidate because it is involved in the inflammation process. Repeated bouts of exercise are known to cause rises in inflammatory markers like TNF. And, since TNF is known to promote fibrosis, the connection between intense endurance exercise and atrial fibrosis and AF vulnerability might involve TNF.

To test the TNF-inflammation link, the researchers did two additional experiments. One was to treat the exercised mice with a TNF blocker, and the other was to study genetically engineered mice without a TNF gene (which rendered them incapable of producing this protein). Remarkably, both these groups of exercised mice did *not* show the atrial remodeling effects, thus strongly suggesting a causative role for TNF and inflammation in promoting atria vulnerable to AF.

We know what you may be thinking: Mice and rats are not people. Of course not, but it is impossible to do these sorts of experiments in humans. For one, the scarring cannot be detected by imaging studies; it was only seen in microscopic examination after the animals were sacrificed. Such methods simply aren't possible in human experiments. But much of science proceeds this way. And more often than not, animal studies produce fascinating and important results.

Human studies

There is, however, evidence of similar effects in humans. Dr. Matthias Wilhelm of the University of Bern, in Switzerland, and his colleagues studied a random sample of 60 runners after a 10-mile running race in Switzerland.[13] They did echocardiograms and signal-averaged ECGs (a special ECG used to calculate electrical properties of the atria) in middle-aged runners. They then compared the measurements with a control group from the general population.

They separated the running group based on lifetime training hours. The Swiss team found that left atrial volume, parasympathetic tone, numbers of premature atrial contractions (PACs), and signal-averaged P-wave duration (a more precise measure of the electrical health of the atria) increased in parallel with lifetime training hours. Although this was a small nonrandomized study with self-reported training hours, the relationship between LA volume (structure) and signal-averaged P-wave duration (electrical) moved in the same direction as the rat-training models.

Inflammation

In the 1990s, some focal arrhythmias required surgery. Italian researchers took advantage of that fact and performed a study in which they did biopsies of the heart in two groups of patients.[14] One group comprised 12 patients with AF not associated with any other diseases such as high blood pressure, diabetes, or heart failure (the type of AF typical of many athletes and which was formerly called "lone AF"). The control group included 11 patients without AF but with the presence of an abnormal conduction pathway between the heart's atria and ventricles called Wolff-Parkinson-White syndrome. The idea was to assess the actual heart muscle for inflammation in patients with AF and those without AF.

Under the microscope, they found that all 12 AF patients had abnormal atrial cells, and more than two-thirds of AF patients had evidence of inflammation. Two patients had patchy areas of atrial scarring. Remember, these patients had no predisposing causes of AF. Yet they had signs of inflammation affecting their atria. These findings suggested a link between inflammation and AF.

Numerous other human studies connect inflammation and AF.[15] Cleveland Clinic researchers compared levels of C-reactive protein (CRP), a marker of inflammation and a predictor of cardiovascular events and stroke, in patients with and without AF.[16] Not only did they observe higher CRP levels in the AF patients, but they also found that patients with a higher incidence of AF had higher CRP levels.

CRP is only one of many markers of inflammation associated with AF in humans. Higher levels of what are called cytokines, including interleukin-6 (IL 6), tumor necrosis factor alpha (TNFα), interleukin 8 (IL-8), and interleukin 10 (IL-10) have all been found to be elevated in patients with AF.[17]

You may be wondering how inflammation can promote AF. The science is not clear about the connection, but one strong hypothesis is that chronic inflammation promotes fibrosis (scarring) in the atria, and that sets the stage for AF.

A simple way to understand inflammation and scarring is to look at the knees or elbows of longtime cyclists. Repeated episodes of road rash have led to the development of scar tissue; the same thing happens to the heart.

In both cases, injury to the skin induces inflammation. White blood cells come to the scene. They secrete chemicals like CRP; TNFα; IL-6, 8, 10; and others. Some of these substances call more cells (chemokines) to the scene, but other chemicals, ones with very long names like matrix metalloproteinase-2 for instance, stimulate the body to make fibrous tissue, or scars.

Scarring might be fine on your elbow, but it's not good in the atria. Remember that electricity in a normal heart flows from cell to cell smoothly. Scar tissue in the atria can disrupt the smooth flow of electrical impulses. That disruption, of course, promotes AF.

The connection to endurance sports

Now you may be thinking, *Okay, I see how inflammation could cause scarring and AF, but how does all this relate to endurance sports?*

This may seem unlikely, but a humanities professor published one of the most compelling papers connecting inflammation, AF, and exercise.[18] Writing in the offbeat journal *Medical Hypothesis*, Dr. Donald Swanson, from the University of Chicago, used a novel computer algorithm to form the hypothesis that excessive endurance exercise, or overtraining, could lead to chronic systemic inflammation that, in turn, could increase the risk of AF.

Swanson conducted a systematic literature-based search for a possible hypothesis connecting AF and exercise. He then used a set of computer programs and processes called Arrowsmith, which is designed to enhance (not replace) human creativity in literature searching. His novel analysis led him to an intriguing review paper in which Lucille Smith, a professor from Appalachian State University, proposed a "cytokine hypothesis of overtraining: a physiological adaptation to excessive stress."[19] Dr. Smith proposed that chronic inflammation is the underlying cause of overtraining syndrome. Repeated muscular and skeletal trauma from intense training results in many local inflammatory reactions. Without adequate time for recovery, all these local inflammation reactions add up to chronic and systemic inflammation.

Most endurance athletes will easily understand her theory: High levels of pro-inflammatory cytokines, such as TNF and IL-6, coordinate a whole-body response that affects three aspects of human biology. (You'll notice they are similar to what happens when we fall ill due to a viral or bacterial infection.)

First, the cytokines communicate with the brain to induce sickness behaviors, such as a depressed mood and fatigue. Being fatigued and depressed make it less likely that we will go out and train, thus promoting healing. Second, high levels of inflammatory cytokines disrupt amino acid regulation, which is vital for maintaining muscle mass and muscle growth. Muscle breakdown and/or slowing of muscle growth are ways in which the body provides for the increased demand for amino acids while repairing chronic inflammation. The overtrained body goes into a catabolic state in which it breaks itself down. Finally, elevated cytokines impair immune function, making an overtrained and inflamed athlete more apt to get ill and, hence, even more inflamed.

Both Swanson and Smith make compelling arguments. Still, these are mostly hypotheses. Let's now move to some actual data.

Hypertrophy and fibrosis

Two scientists from Glasgow, Scotland, aimed to test the theory that heart fibrosis occurs in the hypertrophied muscles of veteran runners. (Remember, scar tissue is the final common pathway of inflammation.)

The two doctors compared 45 elite athletes (older than age 45) with 45 normal sedentary controls.[20]

They made two kinds of measurements: The first were simple measurements of the size of the hearts with an echocardiogram, and the second were blood tests of chemicals known to be part of the matrix of scar tissue (which is collagen).

Not surprisingly, they found that all the athletes had higher degrees of hypertrophy in their hearts. Their key finding, however, was that fibrosis markers were also higher in the veteran athletes, with more hypertrophy leading to higher levels of collagen chemicals. The researchers concluded that there was an association between chemicals that promote heart scarring and the thicker hearts in veteran athletes.

Self-esteem and inflammation

Psychosocial factors clearly affect human health. It's hardly a stretch to say many long-term endurance athletes struggle with their mood and self-esteem. Researchers from London set out to study whether self-esteem might protect against the development of disease by blunting the effects of adrenaline and, yes, you guessed it, inflammation.[21]

They measured self-esteem levels in student volunteers and then exposed them to short periods of mental stress. Their results were provocative. The students with high self-esteem had a smaller increase in heart rate, less decrease in heart rate variability, and fewer inflammatory markers like TNF and IL-6.

Anyone who knows older endurance athletes might recognize the pattern whereby declining performance leads to lower self-esteem and continued training. Both of these responses, it seems, may lead to higher levels of inflammation, fibrosis, and their end result: arrhythmia.

Not all athletes have low self-esteem, certainly. In a fascinating study of Swedish Olympic athletes, researchers studied how competitive anxiety and self-confidence affected self-esteem and perfectionism.[22] They discovered that the relationship between self-esteem and perfectionism differs depending on which dimensions of these characteristics are being considered. Athletes with high self-esteem based on respect and love for themselves had more positive patterns of perfectionism, whereas athletes who have self-esteem that is dependent on being competent at the sport showed a more negative perfectionism. Further, negative patterns of perfectionism related to higher levels of cognitive anxiety and lower levels of self-confidence.

Does lone AF exist?

In the not-too-distant past, patients with AF without an obvious cause—thyroid disease, heart valve disease, or heart failure—were said to have "lone" AF. This label implied that AF occurred for no reason, perhaps due to bad luck.

This old thinking also held that once AF began to occur, it perpetuated itself. The phrase "AF begets AF" became common. In other words, patients with bad luck who got AF for no reason kept having it because AF simply caused more AF.

Maybe you can see the problem with this theory. We've shown you that patients with obesity, high blood pressure, and inflammation—and now endurance athletes—can develop AF. The connecting mechanism is

more subtle than an obvious thyroid or valve problem; it may be inflammation, atrial stretch, or even disorders of the brain-heart connection.

A full discussion of these mechanisms is beyond the scope of this
book, but consider, for instance, that chronic atrial stretch, which could
be seen in patients with obesity or in a chronic endurance athlete—the
atria can't tell the difference—leads to the activation of many pro-fibrotic
(scar-inducing) and hypertrophy-signaling pathways. That is medical-
speak for the process by which heart muscle cells actually transform
into the type of cells (fibroblasts) that lay down collagen or scar tissue in
the atria. This scar tissue then interferes with electrical coupling in the
atria—and boom, you have the milieu for AF.[23]

Recently, a group of AF experts from around the world conducted a
lengthy evidence review and came to the conclusion that the historical
term "lone AF" should be avoided.[24] In short, their take was that AF happens for a reason.

A recent study from an Australian group lends credence to the idea
that AF occurs because of disease in the atria. This group set out to determine whether patients with intermittent AF and no other diseases have
an abnormal atrial substrate. Before we tell you what they found, we
should discuss the stimulus that tipped them off.

The clue came from an important observation made by a famous
group of researchers in Maastricht, in the Netherlands.[25] This group,
led by Dr. Maurits Allessie, studied the progression of AF in an animal
model. After repeatedly inducing AF in goats (they used an implantable pacemaker to cause rapid pacing of the atria, thus inducing AF),
this group made two novel observations: One was that rapid pacing

would induce short runs of AF *and* changes in the electrical properties of the atria. They termed these early and immediate changes the "first factor." Their second finding was that after one to two weeks of continual atrial stimulation, the goats developed persistent AF.

The question, of course, is why did it take weeks to develop persistent AF if electrical changes occurred immediately? This group proposed the presence of a set of second factors[26]—beyond AF alone—that may be responsible for the development and progression of AF. For these second factors, they proposed dilation of the atria, enlargement of the atrial muscle cells, changes in the expression of proteins connecting the cells, and alteration of the matrix holding the cells together. Taken together, they were changes that elicited AF. Later studies confirmed these observations.[27]

Many experts now feel that these structural changes in the atria are what cause AF to persist. After all, if it were solely electrical factors that caused AF, then AF would have appeared immediately in those goats. Instead, it took time.

The structural changes they found are factors we've mentioned previously—fibrosis, dilation, stretch, and inflammation—that also develop in the atria of humans who have high blood pressure, obesity, and sleep apnea. But could these same second factors also be present in the atria of presumably normal people without these diseases?

Now we return to the Australian team that was interested in whether patients with AF and no obvious other diseases had abnormal atria. This group of clinicians did typical catheter-based studies on 25 patients with AF referred for ablation and a control group of 25 patients with left-sided accessory pathways (Wolff-Parkinson-White syndrome, or WPW).[28] People with WPW acted as the control group because WPW is caused by one rogue pathway. The pathway has been present since birth and is not associated with any other heart disease. The research team worked hard to choose AF patients who had no other diseases—no high blood pressure, no diabetes, no valvular disease, just AF.

They found striking differences. Compared with the control group, AF patients had larger left atria and electrical and structural properties consistent with diseased atria. This was a huge surprise because previous thinking was that patients without diseases known to cause AF had healthy atria. The Australian researchers too felt there must be a second factor causing the atria of AF patients to become diseased.

This may have been a small study, but Dr. Allessie himself wrote in an accompanying editorial that the idea of disease in the atria as the cause of AF "may seem rather futuristic, and, in the eyes of some, quite unrealistic and naïve. However, the past decade has shown an unprecedented development in technologies enabling accurate imaging and extensive catheter-based ablation of the atria."[29] Allessie described the development of techniques to diagnose and understand disease in the atria as "crucially important." In other words, if we look hard enough, we will find the reason why people get AF.

We will discuss treatment options for patients with atrial fibrillation in Chapter 8. The association of endurance exercise with AF, its plausibility, and various mechanistic links will feature in the best treatment options. Remember the first rule of medicine: treat the underlying cause, not the symptom.

Ventricular arrhythmia

The same basic principles of triggers (premature beats) and substrate (disorders of smooth conduction in the heart muscle) hold when we discuss ventricular rhythm problems. As we discussed in Chapter 1, the heart rhythm in the ventricle begins with activation of the His-Purkinje network from above (the atria and AV node). In a healthy heart, the signals proceed smoothly from the bundles symmetrically through the ventricular muscle, activating the right and left chambers at the same time.

Recall that the two causes of heart rhythm problems in either atria or ventricles are (1) abnormal automaticity, a fancy medical term for rogue cells acting like pacemaker cells and (2) reentry of electrical impulses through or around barriers to smooth electrical flow. Think short circuits.

Increased automaticity in the ventricles

Premature ventricular complexes (PVCs) or beats are like premature atrial complexes (PACs) or beats in that they begin in a group of rogue cells within the ventricular muscle. These cells act like pacemaker cells and disrupt the normal flow of electricity. PVCs most often occur as single beats. They can, however, string together in runs of fast beats or, in the presence of disease within the muscle, induce short circuits that also result in runs of fast beats. Doctors call this condition ventricular tachycardia (VT, or V-tach).

Reentry in the ventricles

Dilation of the chambers, excess hypertrophy of the muscle, and scar tissue that infiltrates the right and left ventricles can cause the same problems as they do in the atria. These areas act like a big rock in a stream; they set the stage for disruption of the flow of electricity—and arrhythmia.

The link to endurance sports

The evidence linking ventricular arrhythmia and endurance sports is weaker than that for atrial arrhythmia. For one thing, ventricular arrhythmia is less common than atrial arrhythmia, in both the general population and among athletes.

A basic premise of physiology holds that the demands of endurance exercise will exert its effects on both atria and ventricles. In the same way that a bicep grows larger and stronger when exposed to the demands of weight lifting, the heart also adapts to endurance exercise.

One possible reason ventricular arrhythmia is less common than atrial arrhythmia is that the ventricles are less susceptible to these adaptations. Another reason could be purely statistical: namely, AF is more common than ventricular arrhythmia so we see a bigger presence of it in the populations studied.

Ventricular arrhythmia can be more hazardous

In general, atrial arrhythmia is not immediately life-threatening. The same cannot be said for ventricular arrhythmia. While most ventricular arrhythmia in athletes is benign, it is also possible that ventricular arrhythmia may herald the diagnosis of a serious condition of the heart. Premature beats and ventricular tachycardia may be the first signs of diseases such as hypertrophic cardiomyopathy, arrhythmogenic right ventricular dysplasia, or nonischemic cardiomyopathy. Before you run screaming from the room in fear, remember that the seriousness of an arrhythmia depends less on the location of the rogue cells or circuits (atria or ventricle) than on the underlying condition of the heart.

Epidemiologic and observational evidence

In 1982, a Finnish group compared information from ECG monitors worn all day by both 35 highly trained athletes and a control group of nonathletes.[30] They observed slower heart rhythms in athletes, which was not a surprise. They also noted that ventricular arrhythmias were rare in both groups, and not more prevalent in athletes. Similar studies confirmed that PVCs in athletes are uncommon and usually benign.[31]

Italy has a strong tradition of screening athletes for heart problems. In 2002, Dr. Alessandro Biffi and colleagues reported on a study of 355 competitive athletes who had PVCs and complaints of irregular heartbeats.[32] They separated the athletes into three groups based on the number of PVCs per day: Group A comprised 71 subjects with more than 2,000 PVCs per 24-hour period; group B comprised 153 subjects with between 100 and 2,000 PVCs per day; and group C comprised 131 with fewer than 100 PVCs per day. (The heart of the average athlete, you'll recall, beats 80,000 times per day.)

They observed structural heart problems in only 7 percent of the 355 athletes. Moreover, most of these athletes were in the group with the greatest number of PVCs. The researchers then excluded group A athletes from competition. During an average follow-up period of eight years, only one patient—from group A—died suddenly, of arrhythmogenic right ventricular cardiomyopathy while participating in a field hockey game against medical advice.

The authors concluded that frequent ventricular arrhythmias are common in trained athletes and are usually not associated with serious heart disorders. And when ventricular arrhythmias are not associated with heart problems, they do not predict bad outcomes. This group of sports cardiologists proposed that PVCs may be an expression of the "athlete's heart syndrome."

PVCs' response to detraining

To investigate the provocative question of whether training caused the arrhythmia, the Italian researchers did a follow-up in which they evaluated the effect of deconditioning on the 70 remaining athletes from group A who had the highest number of PVCs.[33] When the athletes stopped training and competing, the arrhythmia lessened. PVCs per day dropped from 10,611 to 2,165 (an 80 percent reduction) and runs of non-sustained ventricular tachycardia (NSVT, or PVCs strung together in clusters) per day went from 6 to 0.5 (a 90 percent reduction). In 50 of the 70 athletes, ventricular arrhythmia decreased almost entirely (less than 500 PVCs per 24-hour period and no NSVT). Over the eight-year follow-up, each of the 70 detrained athletes remained free of symptoms.

Complex ventricular arrhythmias

In 2003, Dutch and Belgian cardiologists studied 46 high-level endurance athletes, 80 percent of whom were cyclists, with complex ventricular arrhythmia.[34] That term refers to runs of ventricular tachycardia (VT) rather than just the premature beats of PVCs. Most of these athletes (36 of 46) sought attention because of symptoms such as light-headedness or fainting. That's a key fact to remember as you read their observations.

Unlike the previous reports, this study of symptomatic athletes reported a greater presence of underlying heart problems; definite right ventricular (RV) abnormalities were observed in 59 percent of athletes and suspected in another 30 percent. Eighteen athletes had a major arrhythmic event, nine with cardiac arrest. Disturbingly, the research team could not predict those who had the events based on symptoms and testing.

This 2003 study was the first to suggest that complex ventricular arrhythmias do not necessarily represent a benign finding in endurance athletes. The high prevalence of right ventricular structural and arrhythmic involvement struck the authors as unusual, and soon much more research emerged on the susceptibility of the right ventricle in endurance sports.

Mechanistic and plausibility evidence

A "biomarker" is a medical term for a substance, usually a protein, that can be measured in the blood. Numerous studies have linked an intense and prolonged session of exercise—say a marathon, long-distance triathlon, or bike race—with the release of two commonly used cardiac biomarkers, troponin and BNP.

Troponin is a key protein in the contractile apparatus of the heart muscle cell. Troponin, therefore, belongs inside the muscle cell, not in the blood. In patients who suffer a heart attack, any detectable troponin in the blood indicates injury to the muscle fibers. In a normal person without ongoing heart injury, troponin in the blood is essentially zero. (New high-sensitivity troponin assays can detect tiny amounts of troponin, which may not necessarily indicate heart damage.) This is why doctors consider troponin to be a highly specific marker of heart muscle injury.

Intense and prolonged sessions of exercise can cause a release of troponin into the bloodstream. Intensity, more than duration of the exercise, may be a key factor in troponin release. For instance, the incidence of post-race troponin elevations was lower in ultramarathon finishers than in marathon finishers.[35]

Another factor in troponin release could be the athlete's level of fitness or the presence of underlying heart disease. A study of nonathletic older adults who entered a long-distance walking event found that low-intensity exercise can cause troponin release, especially in those with a heart condition.[36]

No one knows for sure why troponin is released after prolonged exercise. Two possible explanations include an increase in heart muscle permeability (leaky cells) and cell death. Neither sounds good.

BNP stands for "brain natriuretic peptide," which is a small protein released by the ventricles in response to stretch. Unlike troponin, BNP's presence in the blood serves a purpose: When the heart is stretched, BNP acts to reduce the resistance of peripheral blood vessels, and it tells the kidneys to get rid of excess fluid. Doctors call these adjustments "homeostasis," and the human body has a near infinite number of them.

Doctors use BNP to sort out possible causes of breathlessness. For instance, a common cause of breathing problems is congestive heart failure—a condition that leads to volume and/or pressure overload of the ventricles. These patients will have very high levels of BNP. On the other hand, BNP levels will be low when breathlessness is due to pneumonia or asthma.

BNP levels in the blood also rise after exercise.[37] Increases in BNP indicate stretching of or tension in the heart muscle. But unlike troponin increases, which seem more sensitive to intensity, BNP levels appear to depend more on the duration of the exercise. Italian researchers studied nine cyclists competing in the three-week Giro d'Italia and found that BNP levels increased as the race went on, thus correlating with higher energy use over a three-week cycling stage race. This observation may indicate cumulative stress.[38]

Do postexercise biomarker levels increase with damage to the heart?

On this key question, the data conflict. A Canadian group found troponin increases in 14 marathon finishers who also had evidence of impaired RV squeezing (systolic) function and biventricular relaxation (diastolic) abnormalities seen on MRI.[39] That was a bothersome combination—an enzyme known to be released in patients with heart attack correlated with basic heart functioning. The researchers did follow-up MRI scans one week after the race, and no athlete had evidence of heart muscle weakness or scarring. (MRI is currently the most sensitive heart imaging test conducted.)

German researchers found similar results when they studied 105 athletes who performed either a marathon run, one 100-kilometer run, or a mountain-bike marathon. One-third of the athletes showed a significant rise in troponin.[40] This research team chose 21 athletes with elevated troponin levels for a thorough evaluation at three months after the race. By that time, none of the athletes had evidence of structural damage to the RV or LV. One 55-year-old man was noted to have a positive stress test due to a critical blockage in his left main coronary artery—which was likely an incidental finding unrelated to the endurance exercise. Collectively, this example shows how older athletes sometimes get into trouble because of decades of unhealthy living before they took up regular exercise.

In Boston, a group measured biomarkers and performed echocardiogram studies of 60 nonelite runners with an average marathon finish time of four hours.[41] Two-thirds of the athletes had increases in troponin levels, including nearly half with troponin levels over the range indicative of heart attack. The increase in biomarkers correlated with post-race diastolic (relaxation) dysfunction, increased pulmonary pressures (think high blood pressure, but in the lungs), and right ventricular dysfunction (right ventricular mid strain). The novel finding from this study was that training mattered. Well-prepared athletes (measured by weekly mileage before the race) had significantly lower release of biomarkers and less strain as shown on echocardiogram.

Cardiac adaptation to exercise: the upper limit

Most athletes are aware of the strain they put on their heart. Studies on biomarkers make it plain: The stress is enough to cause spillage of a heart muscle protein (troponin) into the blood, and to elevate a chemical used for balancing excess fluid and blood pressure in the body (BNP).

The traditional view of training holds that the heart will respond to training stress by increasing the size of the muscle. In skeletal muscle, this adaptation is called supercompensation, and it results in making the muscle more resilient to future strains.

One question about exercise-induced hypertrophy of the heart is whether it's permanent. Professor Antonio Pelliccia and his colleagues from the Institute of Sports Medicine and Science in Rome studied 40 elite male athletes over a decade.[42] After retirement from sports, most athletes, but not all, showed a decrease in heart dimensions. It's important to note that half of this group had normal measurements in detraining not because of a drop in heart size, but rather because of an increase in body size. (Most cardiac measurements are made relative to body weight.) Additionally, nine athletes (20 percent) continued to show large hearts despite detraining.

These findings—that the heart of an athlete may not return to normal—must be interpreted with caution. We don't know the heart dimensions of these athletes before they began training. It could be that having a big heart is the reason these athletes excelled in sports. But it could be that the persistence of enlargement represents long-term structural change from many years and repeated exposures to micro-injury.

How much remodeling is appropriate? Is there an upper limit at which changes in the heart become inappropriate and even dangerous?

One approach to thinking about the problem of chronic overload comes from valvular heart disease. Patients with leaky aortic or mitral valves do not eject all the blood in one beat; the leaked blood goes back into the pumping chamber. This causes volume overload of the ventricle, which then adapts to this load by gradually dilating. But at some point, the dilation reaches a point at which the heart is damaged beyond repair. Doctors try to operate on patients before they reach this point.

Exercise and the right ventricle

In medical circles, the heart's left ventricle gets most of the attention. When noting the power of the heart, doctors refer to the *left* ventricular ejection fraction (LVEF). That's understandable: The LV is bigger, and it's responsible for delivering blood to the organs and muscles. But the truth is that the right ventricle is equally important. The thinner-walled and smaller RV pumps blood through the lungs for oxygenation. For survival, and for peak sports performance, we need both ventricles to pump strongly and conduct electricity smoothly. The stress of endurance exercise, however, seems to have different effects on the two sides of the heart.

Two Australian sports scientists recently reviewed nearly a hundred scientific studies on the effects of endurance exercise on heart function.[43] They found 14 studies (354 individuals) that included imaging of the heart before and after a session of intense and prolonged exercise. These studies showed a consistent trend: When the heart is imaged after a period of intense, prolonged exercise, the RV dilates and loses power, while the LV remains unaffected.

Two lines of evidence support their conclusions. One is the consistency of the findings. Nearly all the studies these authors reviewed showed similar patterns. There were no outlier studies. A second line of evidence strengthening the notion of increased RV susceptibility to endurance exercise lies in the findings of two separate studies that found a correlation between postexercise biomarkers and RV dysfunction.[44] What's more, a study in late 2016 of endurance trail runners whose hearts were examined with state-of-the-art ultrasound during and after a race confirmed the enhanced right ventricle's susceptibility to exercise.[45]

Of course, we need to be careful here. The observation of greater RV susceptibility to exercise is intriguing and suggestive, but the rules of medical evidence apply: Observing something (transient RV dysfunction after exercise) does not necessarily mean exercise causes damage to the heart. Observational evidence is not as strong as randomized trials because of selection bias and possible confounding factors.

That said, given that ventricular arrhythmia is the underlying cause of most cases of sudden death in athletes, these observations warrant further thought. Is it plausible, for instance, that the RV would be the weak link? And if the RV is susceptible to damage from exercise, could that have long-term consequences?

Possible causes of RV susceptibility

Let's consider two reasons why the RV may be susceptible to damage from exercise. The first lies in the physics of exercise. The demands of exercise lead to higher blood pressure, both in the peripheral arteries and in the pulmonary artery (the conduit from the heart to the lungs). Increasing levels of blood pressure (or greater resistance to blood flow) inhibit delivery of blood. Medical people call the resistance to flow in the peripheral arteries "systemic vascular resistance" (SVR), and the resistance to flow in the lung arteries "pulmonary vascular resistance" (PVR).

The catch here for the RV is that during exercise we can only reduce our PVR by 30 to 50 percent, while SVR can drop by 75 percent.[46] Training does not improve our ability to reduce resistance to blood flow in the lungs. Training does, however, lead to an increased ability to pump higher blood volumes. So more flow and less elasticity in the pulmonary artery means that athletes can develop higher peak pulmonary artery pressures, meaning that their RV feels a greater increase in wall stress than the LV.

The second line of support for RV susceptibility comes from animal studies. The same group of researchers from Montreal who did the elegant rodent studies on exercise and AF had previously teamed with a Spanish group to study ventricular arrthymias. In their famous "marathon rat" study,[47] the researchers compared highly exercised rats to sedentary control rats. The "marathon rats" developed an increased susceptibility to induced ventricular arrhythmias, RV chamber dilation, and weakness and enhanced scarring within the ventricles, which the researchers assessed by autopsy after the experiment. Ventricular tachycardia could be induced in 5 of 12 exercised rats (42 percent) and only 1 of 16 sedentary rats (6 percent). To support the observation of exercise-induced scarring in trained rats, the researchers also found higher levels of multiple proteins that signal scar formation in the exercising group.

Why do these observations add up to more than an academic argument about ventricles? Because of the idea that endurance exercise could cause conditions (scarring and chamber enlargement) in which life-threatening ventricular arrhythmias are plausible.

To explain, we need to briefly delve into a rare disease called arrhythmogenic right ventricular cardiomyopathy (ARVC). Patients with ARVC suffer from repetitive bouts of ventricular arrhythmia that most often originate from patches of scar tissue and fatty infiltration of the right ventricle. In slightly more than half the cases, ARVC has a strong heritable nature, passed down through families.

Italian researchers from the Veneto region first discovered that young athletes with ARVC had a fivefold greater risk of dying from it than non-athletes with ARVC.[48] At the time, the idea that endurance exercise made a heart condition worse, not better, was big news in the medical world. Giving credence to their provocative observation connecting exercise and worse outcomes in ARVC was the fact that a pre-participation screening program that restricted participation of affected athletes reduced the rate of ARVC-associated deaths.

Why would exercise make RV disease worse? Think about the underlying defect in ARVC: Most (but not all) of those afflicted patients have heritable mutations in the genes that code for desmosomes, which are mechanical bridges linking one heart cell to the next. As you remember from Chapter 1, a functional heart rhythm depends on healthy cell-to-cell connections. If exercise puts mechanical stress on the connections between heart cells via an increase in stretch and wall stress, people with ARVC who exercise intensely develop even more disruption of cells, which leads to patches of scar and fatty infiltration, and more chance of arrhythmia.

Now you ask, how does this rare disease apply to the average endurance exerciser? So far we can only speculate, but some sports scientists feel that intense exercise performed over sufficiently long periods can cause an ARVC-type disease, perhaps only in susceptible individuals.

The theory got started with the 2003 Dutch and Belgian study mentioned earlier of 46 athletes. The athletes in this study all presented with ventricular arrhythmias, which, in nearly all cases, originated from the RV. Because only one of the 46 athletes had a family history of arrhythmia, the authors coined the term "exercise-induced ARVC."

In 2010, this group published a gene study of a different group of athletes with ventricular arrhythmia that bolstered the exercise-induced ARVC theory.[49] In that study, the research team did MRI scans and gene studies in 47 different athletes with right ventricle VT. (Doctors can easily tell the origin of the VT by assessing its appearance on a standard ECG. If the VT has a left bundle branch [LBB] pattern, it's usually an RV source; if the VT has a right bundle branch [RBB] pattern, it's from the LV.) On MRI, more than 75 percent of these athletes had evidence of ARVC. The key part of this study was the genetic analysis. Remember, half the people with ARVC harbor genetic mutations in desmosomal proteins. So, if exercise had nothing to do with damaging the right ventricle, the researchers would have expected about half of the athletes to have this mutation.

But only 6 of 47 (12.8 percent) athletes in their series had a known ARVC mutation. That was much lower than expected. What is more, no mutations were found in the 20 athletes performing more than average amounts of weekly exercise, yet all met the criteria for definite or suspected ARVC. These findings, therefore, supported the idea that an ARVC-like disease could be acquired through intense exercise without an identifiable genetic susceptibility. In 2012, this group wrote a review paper summing up the evidence for their hypothesis.[50]

The problem with this hypothesis is that it comes from only one group of researchers. Independent replication makes scientific and medical findings stronger.

In 2014, a group of researchers at Johns Hopkins University published a study that lent support to the provocative hypothesis.[51] Johns Hopkins has a large referral program in which they follow hundreds of patients with known ARVC. In this study, they compared the exercise history of ARVC patients with and without mutations in the genes that affect desmosomes. They called the disease in ARVC patients without gene mutations "gene-elusive" ARVC.

Their findings were clear and compelling: Every one of the gene-elusive patients were endurance athletes. Moreover, gene-elusive patients who had done the most intense exercise prior to presentation had a younger age of presentation, a greater likelihood of having all the criteria for ARVC, and were more likely to have a ventricular arrhythmia in follow-up.

A year earlier, in another groundbreaking study from the Johns Hopkins group, the researchers first observed that the amount and intensity of exercise increased the likelihood of diagnosis, ventricular arrhythmia, and development of heart failure among people who were mutation carriers for ARVC.[52] In this study, they recruited 87 people from their series who either had ARVC or were carriers of the mutations known to cause the disease. The latter group were family members of individuals who had already been diagnosed with ARVC. The researchers observed striking findings: Symptoms of the disease (arrhythmias) developed in endurance athletes at a younger age (30 versus 40 years old on average). The greater the duration and intensity of exercise, the greater was the presentation of the disease. Thirteen individuals in this series suffered cardiac arrest; all were endurance athletes.

This observation was important because it showed that exercise promoted and worsened a life-threatening disease in at least a proportion of genetically susceptible mutation carriers. Dr. Calkins and his colleagues called it the "double-hit hypothesis"[53] in that for some people, it took both a gene mutation and endurance exercise to cause the disease.

A colleague told me she works with a family in which two siblings have a desmosomal mutation typical of ARVC. One is an endurance athlete who has had multiple episodes of VT and is treated with an internal defibrillator. The other, a couch potato, has a perfect rhythm and a heart that appears to function normally. Both have the genetic basis for the disease (genotype), but only the athlete has the disease (phenotype).

Summary of evidence

Taken together, these data from two separate groups of researchers suggest that exercise can in some cases promote severe disease in the right ventricle. Physics studies and animal data confirm and render plausible the idea that the RV is more susceptible than the LV. Clinical studies on mutation carriers for proteins responsible for connecting cells show that exercise can induce or worsen disease in the RV.

The thinking behind Phidippides cardiomyopathy is that enough endurance exercise can cause heart muscle disease in the ventricle. It clearly can in the small number of patients with desmosomal mutations like those seen in ARVC. There are also very small numbers of susceptible individuals who have gene-elusive ARVC in which endurance exercise is the "second-hit" that causes muscle disease.

It all sounds scary, but there are crucial caveats. For one thing, these are highly selected groups of athletes (or family members of athletes) who presented with symptoms. They represent only a tiny fraction of elite athletes. The vast majority of endurance athletes do not develop severe ventricular arrhythmias.

The connection between endurance exercise and ventricular arrhythmia will require much more research. In the next chapter, we will explore what sort of symptoms to look for in yourself.

Athletes and coronary artery disease

In older adults, a common cause of heart rhythm problems is blockages in the blood supply to the heart. This is known as coronary artery disease. My medical partner humorously compares the practice of cardiology with caring for your house: if both the electricity and plumbing are not working, you fix the toilet first.

Mountains of evidence support the notion that exercise protects against (and treats) standard atherosclerotic heart disease, or hardening of the arteries. In fact, doctors prescribe cardiac rehabilitation programs for patients who have had bypass surgery after a heart attack. Evidence suggests these exercise-centered programs improve outcomes. Yet cardiologists rarely feel surprise when an older athlete presents with a blockage in his or her coronary arteries.

It's true that regular exercise favors health, but it is also true that vigorous exercise greatly increases the short-term risk of coronary events— up to 16-fold in one huge study of male physicians.[54] In Chapter 2, we noted that the underlying cause of sudden events on the sports field turns on age; in patients older than 35, the most likely cause is coronary events.

It's a paradox. Regular low- or moderate-intensity exercise reduces the burden of the risk factors that associate with coronary artery disease.

Exercisers, for instance, have better blood pressure, diabetes less often, favorable cholesterol profiles, and, usually, less obesity. It makes perfect sense, therefore, that those who exercise as a hobby would be inoculated against heart disease. But medical practice rarely follows the rules.

In 1979, Professor Tim Noakes, a running guru at the University of Capetown, South Africa, and author of the best-selling book *The Lore of Running*, and his colleagues published a five-case autopsy series of accomplished distance runners (ages 27 to 44). All five had moderate to severe coronary disease.[55] Two of the five patients died as a result of abrupt blockage of a coronary artery—a myocardial infarction or heart attack. Three deaths were accidental: in two of these cases, severe coronary disease was observed, and in one, a 27-year-old with a smoking history, doctors noted both moderate coronary disease and fatty infiltration in the RV and scar tissue in the LV.

When discussing the limits of autopsy studies, the authors wrote something relevant to the topic of this book: "Our data also do not exclude the possibility that marathon running hastened their deaths."

A few small, more recent studies raise the idea that long-term endurance training might promote atherosclerosis in predisposed people. In 2008, for example, a research group from Essen, Germany, took advantage of the ability of CT scans to detect calcium deposits in coronary arteries and MRI scans to see scar tissue.[56] These technologies allow doctors to see the actual hardening of the arteries (the calcium buildup) and the scarring. The researchers recruited 108 marathon runners over the age of 50 to study the prevalence of coronary artery calcium in relation to established risk factors, and to study the role of coronary calcium in causing heart damage or acute events.

These were not one-time marathoners. Participants in this study had completed at least five full-distance marathons in the preceding three years and had no known health problems. The researchers graded the risk of heart disease with a multicomponent scoring system called the Framingham Risk Score (FRS). They used a comparison group of nonrunners who were matched by age, body mass index, and FRS.

(The Framingham study is a famous longitudinal cohort study in which residents of the Massachusetts town have been followed for decades. It is the study that first showed how risk factors such as blood pressure, diabetes, and high cholesterol increased the risk for heart disease.)

Their findings were intriguing. Runners had a lower FRS (fewer risk factors for heart disease) but did not have lower amounts of coronary calcium than age-matched controls. In fact, the opposite was true: When compared with FRS-matched controls, marathon runners had triple the amount of coronary calcium. Triple! The degree of calcium and the number of marathons run predicted the presence of scar tissue found on MRI scans. Overall, 12 percent of the runners had evidence of ventricular scarring versus 3 percent of the control group. During a short follow-up period of less than two years, four runners with high calcium scores experienced coronary events.

One caveat of this study is that many of the runners in this series were former smokers, including 5 percent who continued to smoke while training. (*Who smokes while training?*) And, in a review article, sports scientist Dr. André La Gerche noted that "it would seem that many of the subjects studied had only fairly recently taken up marathon running, which introduces the potential for a selection bias in which subjects concerned about their previous or current health status might be more likely to volunteer for a 'screening' study."[57]

In a follow-up study in which these same athletes were followed for six years, the research team found no increased risk of heart attack or death rate in the runners compared to a matched population.[58]

A smaller study of 25 finishers of the Minneapolis marathon showed similar findings.[59] Again, the research team used CT scans to compare the degree of atherosclerosis of marathon runners versus an age-matched control group of nonathletes. The marathon group had a lower resting heart rate, a lower BMI, and better HDL (good) cholesterol. Yet the research team observed significantly more calcified plaque in the marathon group (mean, 274 mm^3 versus 169 mm^3).

To complicate matters here, cardiologists continue to debate the importance of calcified plaque seen on CT scans, as most acute events like heart attack come from soft, noncalcified plaque. In fact, one study of CT scans and statin use showed that cholesterol-lowering drugs decreased the chance of cardiac events even though patients on the drugs had higher degrees of coronary calcification.[60]

Taken together, these studies also reveal yet another exercise paradox. On paper, marathon runners boast healthier numbers and have lower heart rates, smaller body sizes, and better cholesterol numbers, but their coronary arteries look like those of an average couch potato or cigarette smoker.

We can't draw conclusions from these small observational studies, but it's hard not to be at least a little concerned. One theory for increased coronary calcium in runners may be that the repetitive pounding of running causes the skeleton to leach calcium, which may then accumulate in the coronary arteries. Interestingly, there are no publications of coronary calcium in endurance athletes who do different sports.

Dr. La Gerche suggests another possible idea. "Atherosclerosis," he says, "does not disappear when running shoes are put on for the first time." He suggests a better study might be to look at lifelong exercise enthusiasts. It's possible that those who have maintained a healthy life-style for decades may not harbor the same amount of coronary calcium.[61]

In early 2015, a research paper from Denmark garnered significant attention in the lay press because it boldly concluded there was a U-shaped association of running and death rate.[62] That is, light and moderate joggers had lower death rates than sedentary controls, but strenuous joggers had death rates similar to the sedentary controls. This paper, with its common-sense conclusions, suffered from a severe statistical problem: The group of vigorous runners included only 36 of more than 1,000 runners in the study. Although the authors reported that vigorous runners had nearly twofold higher death rates, the confidential intervals were wide, ranging from a 50 percent lower death rate all the way up to an eightfold *higher* death rate. You simply cannot draw any conclusions from this sort of data.

Let's conclude this section with a study that provides perspective on the overall safety of marathons. In 2012, a large group of US sports scientists performed a massive registry study of nearly 11 million participants in marathons and half-marathons over a 10-year period.[63]

Get this: Only 59 runners suffered cardiac arrest during the race. That's an incidence of 0.54 per 100,000. Most of these cases were of cardiovascular causes, either from hypertrophic cardiomyopathy or coronary artery disease. The authors concluded that "marathons and half-marathons are associated with a low overall risk of cardiac arrest and sudden death." We feel confident in modifying the low risk of events by calling it a *damn* low risk of cardiac events.

The evidence presented in this chapter suggests a clear link between endurance exercise and heart rhythm disorders. Population studies show that endurance exercise increases the risk of AF; animal and human studies support that evidence. The finding that a reduction in training intensity and/or length often fixes the problem further bolsters the connection between prolonged exercise and heart damage. Additionally, imaging studies indicate that inflammation, scarring, and stretching frequently take place in the athletic heart.

While the findings on damage to the ventricles of endurance athletes are less conclusive, the evidence still suggests a connection between the strain placed on the heart by endurance exercise and the onset of arrhythmia, particularly in the right ventricle.

As similar evidence continues to accumulate, additional research will eventually help us confirm and understand these links. Meanwhile, there's the practical question of how to look for warning signs in yourself and what to do about them. We'll address those questions in the following chapters.

CASE STUDY
Mike Endicott: Ventricular tachycardia
Diagnosed at age 50

CHRIS CASE

Mike Endicott was always interested in endurance sports, even when he was a teenager. He hiked the Appalachian Trail in 1973 when he was 18 years old. He moved to Boulder, Colorado, in 1980, to take advantage of the climbing opportunities in the area. Though he came as a rock climber, he soon became a fan of trail running.

"By nature I'm a person who likes to train. I race to train; a lot of people train to race. [Racing] was kind of anti-climactic. I use racing as kind of a gauge as to where you're at, but I much prefer to be just out doing stuff. I just like the movement and activity, being outside," Endicott says.

His interests evolved again, so that six months of the year he would be Nordic skiing and the other six months would be devoted to riding road and mountain bikes. He was moving nonstop.

He was an independent sales representative, managing sales in Colorado, Utah, Wyoming, and New Mexico, in the cycling and outdoor sports industries. A typical day might include a fine mix of work and play. If he was working in Moab, he might take much of the day off to do a solo ride along the White Rim Trail, a

100-mile epic mountain bike ride through Canyonlands National Park. Then he'd eat, go into town, and make his work visits. Then he'd drive to Salt Lake City and get ready for the next morning. He was working seven days a week.

"I was burning the candle at both ends. I was having a ball. I was working, I was making a good living, but, boy, was I burning it and I didn't realize it," Endicott says now. The result was that any racing Endicott did would be hit or miss, solid or so-so.

"A good coach would have told me, 'Oh, I know what's going on.' It was classic: I was chronically overtrained. That was the beginning of what probably caused all my issues. Probably. Likely. Nobody will ever know, but that's a likely cause: chronic overtraining," he says.

Endicott lived this way for years. He'd ski a marathon race in Yellowstone on Saturday, then drive to Steamboat and do another marathon on Sunday. He loved it. And he was able to work in between.

"It's not good for you though," he says, looking back at his life now. "But who would know? You would think it's good for you."

Then, one day in 2005, he headed to Devil's Thumb, a Nordic ski area in the Fraser Valley of Colorado. "I had created the perfect storm over a good 20-year period, but it all came to a head here because of the week or two prior to this race," he said.

Before heading to Devil's Thumb, Endicott had been in Boston at a sales meeting. Immediately after the sales meeting, he returned to Colorado and went straight to Breckenridge to do a ski race. He had a mediocre race, a "spit-blood race," one that hurt. He then drove straight to Steamboat Springs to conduct clinics, throwing in an interval workout and feeling good.

He hadn't slept well the night before heading to Devil's Thumb, and he knew he was tired. But, like so many of us, he just liked being out there. He felt he needed to get into shape, since it was early season, and this would be good for his form.

He didn't eat much before the race except for two big Starbucks coffees. An hour from the start, he downed a few caffeinated Gu packs. It was cold, around zero degrees, overcast, with light snow falling and a bit of a breeze swirling 'round. All of the ingredients for the perfect storm were in place.

"I'm having a good race, and probably about a third of the way through, I could see the people I wanted to reel in. . . . I was having fun, going after it," he says. "I saw one little nice rise and thought, 'OK, I'll punch up this thing' because there was a guy right in front of me that I wanted to reel in. We were always humorously competitive. Punched up over this rise and all of a sudden, I don't feel good, something's not right. Something was beating inside my chest. No pain, no discomfort, but I was a little dizzy."

Endicott stopped to catch his breath. He was hyperventilating. As he stood beside the trail, people started to pass him. Friends asked if he was okay. He told them he'd be all right. He told himself to keep going because he just couldn't figure out what was happening. He tried to ski. He wasn't racing any longer, as most of the field had passed him by, but he skied on.

He felt like he was drunk. He could hardly stay up on his legs; he would collapse and get back up, his heart still doing something strange inside his chest.

"I knew something was bad. I knew the race was over. It was survival mode: 'I got to get back to the lodge,'" he says. "Luckily, I knew it was mostly downhill so I got off the racecourse, which was a mistake in retrospect."

By the time the last skiers had passed by, Endicott was done; he collapsed in the snow and began to die. He was on his back, barely maintaining consciousness, in a skin suit, in the snow, in zero-degree weather. There was no pain, but he couldn't catch his breath. He tried to yell for help, but he could barely make a noise; he could only wave his pole.

"Fairly quickly I realized I'm in deep shit here. Basically I figured I was done, this was it," he says. "It's interesting . . . at the time, my emotions were . . . I was frustrated. It was not on my list of things to do because I was kind of a type A, my dog was in my truck, we were going to go out and do a ski when I was done, I had work to do that afternoon, phone calls to make. It just wasn't on my list of things to do—to die on the ski trails. I was pissed [laughs]. I was beating on my chest with my hands saying, 'Come on, something's got to work here.' So I struggled in and out of consciousness out there in the snow for about an hour. I don't know how long I was out, and then I'd come back again, and then I'd try to look around and then I'd get dizzy again. It was ugly."

By pure chance, two of his friends went out for a cooldown after their race and the awards ceremony. They saw Mike wave his arm out of the corner of their eyes and skied to find a fallen friend dying in the snow.

As they snowmobiled Mike out on a sled, he was belligerent, trying to fight whatever it was he was going through.

"I was just fighting the whole thing, pissing and moaning, yelling, just thinking this is stupid; this is not what you would expect," he says. "I was even swinging at my buddies, saying, 'This is ridiculous!'"

Mike was in ventricular tachycardia. The result was sudden cardiac arrest. He was 50. It sounds grave, and it was, but by his own admission, it was a miracle he survived.

Doctors ruled out any plumbing issues in Endicott's heart. Had he visited a clinic the day before the race, it's more than likely that nothing would have shown up on paper, on any test, that would have led the doctors to stop him from racing.

"They would have pronounced me healthy as a horse," he says. "The ECG would have been perfect because I wasn't having any symptoms. Nothing was symptomatic whatsoever. No PVCs, no weird rhythms. Everything on paper [was fine], with the exception of the little bit of artery disease—not much more than a lot of people that age."

After looking at a lot of different cases and talking to a number of doctors, Endicott came to a conclusion: "I did all this to myself—by personality. And if someone had come to me before this happened—and this is a key part of reality—and said you need to back off because this is your future, would I have changed anything? Probably not. I would likely do the same activities, but I would rest and recover more. Just because that's the nature of a lot of us. We enjoy doing it, we're probably doing it too much, we're selfish about it, and we're going to be in denial, and that's a problem that a lot of these electrophysiologists have when we ask 'Why me?'"

One of the problems with a lot of athletes—the problem with Endicott—is that they can't stop asking why. How could this happen to me, someone who has built his life around being active? It just didn't make sense. Endicott was in denial, even after it happened. But he wasn't unique. The most difficult component to life after heart malfunction, for many, is the psychological struggle.

He and others like him are desperate to know what went wrong. They want the cardiologist to help solve the puzzle. But doctors will not speculate. The doctor's job is to stabilize patients, keep them alive, and try to give them quality of life.

In Endicott's case, that meant having three failed ablations before a fourth successful attempt. Because his was exercise-induced tachycardia, he would not only be awake for the procedure, but would be caffeinated and given intravenous adrenaline to improve the chances of inducing arrhythmia while he was on the table. Catheters were sent through his femoral veins and arteries, on both sides, and led into the heart. For his first attempt, he lay awake for eight hours; it failed to identify the source of the arrhythmia.

For the next attempt, doctors at the University of Oklahoma, one of the most experienced facilities in the United States, tried for sixteen hours to locate the culprit tissue. Still, they couldn't induce tachycardia.

"It was a brutal session. It was endurance. But they couldn't find a focal point. So they did some burns; both times they burned some places where they thought the problem was," Endicott says.

Though his doctors believed they had ablated the problem, within the next few months Endicott was experiencing episodes again. Yes, stubborn as he was, Endicott was going out and doing the things he loved to do. And, yes, this was leading to more episodes of V-tach. Eventually, it was determined that his condition was too perilous not to insert an implantable cardio-verter defibrillator (ICD). Life carried on.

The ICD can be a beautiful device, shocking the heart back into rhythm, saving a life from the inside out. But it isn't with-out its discomforts. It is, according to Endicott, like getting hit by lightning. If you're on a bike when it happens, it's going to knock you off. If you're standing up, it's going to drop you to the floor. It's a very quick shock. It determines that the rhythm of your heart is out of synch, it determines what kind of rhythm you need, and then it instantaneously reboots you. Your heart actu-ally stops so it can restart the right way.

It may sound like a miracle, and it can be. But it can also lead to catastrophe, in what is called an electrical storm. Endi-cott suffered such a storm when he was performing as a mem-ber of a band at a retirement community. His instrumental solo bumped his level of adrenaline and he went into V-tach.

"I would go into V-tach, I would get the shock [from the ICD], and the shock would convert me into sinus rhythm for a couple of beats, but there was so much adrenaline that I would get thrown right back into V-tach," Endicott says. "It was a cycle, and it was brutal. It's going to do its job until I'm dead."

The folks gathered around him didn't know what was happening. He was able to hide his embarrassment by slowly leaving the area where the concert was taking place, finally curling up in a ball on the floor in another part of the community. He had only one to one-and-a-half minutes between shocks. When the paramedics arrived he was still convulsing. They weren't able to detect a heartbeat, so external defibrillation was used to return his heart to a normal sinus rhythm. He was lucky. He had suffered through 32 consecutive shocks from the ICD.

"We're talking about something that feels like 1,000 volts. It happens quickly but you'll see a flash. . . . It was basically like being tortured," he says. The result was an acute case of post-traumatic stress disorder (PTSD). It was something that Endicott never knew anything about until it was upon him. He was rewired, yet again. Little things in life, as happens with PTSD, became too much to deal with—beyond-category climbs, as he puts it. It took him two years to recover.

Finally, in 2009, he was referred to the cardiology department at Brigham and Women's Hospital in Boston. Their top electrophysiologist, Dr. William Stevenson, reviewed the case and decided to try one more ablation. This time the procedure was performed on the outside surface of his heart. It worked—after a four-hour examination.

"If I read a story like this I wouldn't believe you. I would be in denial because I love doing things like this. I still try to find ways to be able to do things like this and I've been through the wringer," Endicott says. "I've gotten a little smarter about it. But I'm also practical and pragmatic and I could always see the humor in it, even when I was lying in the snow and I knew I was likely not going to survive. I didn't think I was going to make it. There were no white lights for me. I was scared and I was coming out of being clinically dead. I even had to laugh to myself and say what a waste. 'I'm here lying in the snow . . . at least I'll be well preserved [laughs].' But I was very frustrated because of that lack of control."

The complexity of the heart, the body, human physiology, and genetics makes it extremely difficult to predict when and in which heart something catastrophic like this will take place. Why did this happen to Endicott when it did? Well, there are 50 years of cumulative variables that would need to be considered to fully understand what went wrong on that cold, crisp day at Devil's Thumb.

Some of it is genetic. Did he have a tendency toward higher blood pressure? Yes. What about cholesterol? He was always well below average for that, like many athletes with a healthy diet. Plaque buildup? A little, but nothing out of the ordinary. These are the little clues that would be easy to dismiss, but combined with his stressful lifestyle, filled with epic endurance events and a somewhat frantic employment schedule—the acquired stressors that this chapter shows can lead to arrhythmia—they sketch a picture of an impending storm on the distant horizon. Add stress and cold weather, and that picture quickly became an IMAX 3D feature film on dying in the woods, alone.

"For years it was like the hints were there in all the studies, and [researchers] always conclude that more research needs to be done. And they're still saying that," Endicott says. "I've done the research, folks. It happened to me. I've had friends that are either dead or alive that it happened to. The research is out there; listen to it. Now they're finally starting to acknowledge those facts and those examples that something is going on."

5 | What to look for in yourself

EVERYONE'S DIFFERENT, but my case of atrial fibrillation (AF) is instructive about what athletes may face. It happened to me at age 48. I was training hard for the upcoming summer bike race season. My team and I were putting in long training miles, race efforts, and threshold work. We were racing on the weekends and training during the week.

Then I broke my ribs in a crash. If you have ever broken a rib, you know how much the injury slows you down. Breathing hurts, sleeping hurts, and sneezing is like an electrical shock coursing through your body.

But there was a third component that led to my AF. On top of an intense training load and a rib injury, I was also working full-time as an electrophysiologist. It's fascinating work, but it's also exhausting; among other things, it involves standing in the laboratory draped in a heavy lead apron for hours at a time, walking repeatedly down the long halls of the hospital, and continuing to make patient rounds. Being a cardiologist is demanding in itself, but with a rib injury and fatigue, it was fertile ground for the development of AF.

One hot summer day after the crash, I was on a training ride with my teammates. That day I had taken no pain meds, and my ribs hurt a lot on the ride. But I was doing okay. I was rotating in the line, taking my turns. Then it happened. We were 40 kilometers from home when I noticed an abrupt onset of breathlessness and an utter loss of power. It was more than the heat; it was something else. My heart rate monitor showed funny numbers. The beats were irregular, and any slight rise in the pavement caused my heart rate to spike much higher than normal.

I had to let the ride go on without me. Moments before, I was pulling through easily. But now I couldn't hang with the group. A friend stayed with me, pushing me up hills. When I finally got home, I told my wife that I thought I was in AF. She is a hospice and palliative care doctor, so for her, AF is hardly alarming. She felt my pulse and seconded my suspicion. "You have an irregularly irregular pulse," she said. "Yep, you have AF."

Since I am a cardiologist, I decided to confirm the diagnosis myself. I showered and dressed and went to my office to do an ECG, an echocardiogram, and some simple blood tests to check my thyroid function. The tests showed that my heart was fine, other than the rhythm being in AF. That night, I went home and rested. My partner in our practice called in some medication for me. I swallowed the pills and went to bed preparing myself mentally for a day of tolerating the fibrillation and irregular pulse. I figured I'd do a full day of work and then get cardioversion (shock) afterward.

The next morning, I woke up without the butterfly sensations in my chest. My pulse was regular. I was back in sinus rhythm, and I felt a small hope that I was in the clear.

I took Flecainide (a drug to stabilize heart rhythm) for a few months, a regimen I prescribe for my patients. My heart improved, but it wasn't exactly smooth sailing. Over the next year or so, I experienced frequent skips, jumps, and flutters (doctors label them "palpitations") of the heart rhythm. I could feel them in my chest and throat. They occurred at rest and when I rode. On two other occasions in the following months, I had a few hours of AF episodes.

In retrospect, I should have seen the signs. I was injured, I was training excessively in the heat of summer, and I was still trying to work full time. What I should have been looking for was balance; it should have been obvious I was asking too much of my body. Instead, I kept pushing myself to continue my routine—my "normal." But of course I was anything but normal by then.

Warning symptoms

If my case has any instructive use, it should be to demonstrate that there are plenty of warning signs of trouble. The key is to heed them. But what are they? And what should you be looking for in yourself?

There are two types of symptoms to worry about. Both fall into the category of "not normal." Your immediate sensations are a good guide. You have probably been training for many years, if not most of your life. Those years of training have given you a good sense of what "normal" feels like. What you are looking for is anything that falls outside the boundaries of normal. For example, a brief flutter in your chest on a ride is probably nothing; nearly everyone gets one from time to time. A flutter that won't go away, however, is cause for concern. A sustained irregular heartbeat is an abnormal feeling that should set off an alarm.

Sensations that are not normal include

- Racing heart: any sustained racing of the heart that won't go away.

- Chest pressure or pain, especially pressure or pain that worsens during exertion.

- Labored breathing: difficult breathing that is out of proportion to effort (everyone breathes hard when climbing hills or sprinting).

- Fainting or near-fainting: anything more serious than the everyday lightheadedness you might feel after a hard effort.

These symptoms are serious warning signs that should alert you to possible trouble. Sustained chest pressure or chest pain warrants a call to 911. All others warrant an appointment with your doctor, sooner rather than later. If you experience these symptoms, you should stop training until you can be evaluated by a professional.

Secondary warning signs include sensations that are not normal but usually less worrisome, including

- Palpitations: skips, jumps, or flutters of the heart rhythm.

- Consistently low power: A decrease in sustainable power is the real warning sign here. There are lots of reasons for low power output, including natural variability, overtraining, and medical conditions. Usually it's the first two. But if your sustainable power drops, take note.

- Excess fatigue: Like low power, generalized fatigue can be caused by many factors. In fact, fatigue may be one of medicine's most nonspecific symptoms. Causes range from poor sleep or overtraining to a host of specific medical conditions.

- Excess irritability: Irritability is often a sign of overtraining or inadequate nutrition, but patients with arrhythmia or other medical conditions often say they are irritable. Spouses sometimes notice this symptom first.

When should you see a doctor?

Sustained racing of the heart, chest pain, difficulty breathing, or fainting are symptoms that mandate a formal evaluation by a doctor. The four less specific symptoms mentioned above—palpitations, low power, excess fatigue, excess irritability—may warrant a doctor's visit, too. But those symptoms are less worrisome.

Before you see a doctor, try some simple things first. Skips of the heart rhythm, low power, fatigue, and irritability often improve with rest and nutrition. Although many athletes find any period without exercise challenging, either a short period of rest or an even longer period of prolonged rest may resolve the symptoms.

Another thing an athlete with the less worrisome symptoms can do before going to the doctor is to pay close attention to nutrition. This means not only eating enough healthy food, but also abstaining from the following irritants to the heart.

Alcohol

By far, the number one (legal) irritant to the heart is alcohol. The relationship of alcohol to heart rhythm is well known. The French paradox suggests that one or two drinks per day may lower the risk of heart disease, but the relationship of alcohol to arrhythmia is linear, as shown in Figure 5.1. One drink per day leads to a small risk of AF; two drinks double the risk; three drinks triple the risk; and so on. Numerous studies have confirmed that reducing alcohol intake may reduce the burden of arrhythmia.

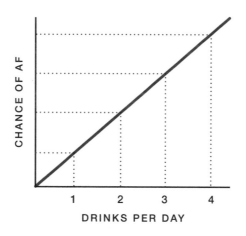

FIGURE 5.1. Alcohol consumption and the risk of arrhythmia[1]

Stress

Excess stress, whether mental (trying to juggle an overbooked calendar) or emotional (divorce or the death of a loved one), can associate with heart rhythm problems. Yet it is impossible to be alive and not experience stress. The issue is not avoidance of stress, but how well you manage it.

I've helped hundreds of patients through arrhythmia flare-ups caused in large part by major life events. Quite often, there is little that you can do to avoid these things. What you can keep in mind, however, is the knowledge that the stress will pass, and so may the burst of arrhythmia. If you are experiencing some of the less worrisome symptoms of trouble mentioned above, one option you have before seeing the doctor is to let some time pass until you clear the immediate cause of stress.

However, chest pain, breathlessness, sustained racing of the heart, or fainting should not be passed off as stress. These more severe symptoms warrant attention.

Caffeine

Oddly enough, caffeine's relationship to rhythm problems is unclear. Old thinking had it that caffeine could cause or exacerbate rhythm problems. New data, including multiple large observational studies, suggest that caffeine does not associate with arrhythmias. In fact, the most provocative finding indicates that the favorite pick-me-up of so many athletes may actually confer a lower risk of arrhythmia. That's not a misprint. It may sound strange, but it's what the science shows. Here are a few of the largest studies on caffeine and heart disease:

Caffeine and premature beats. In the largest study to evaluate the
association of dietary patterns and heart rhythm problems, a group of US
researchers published a report from the Cardiovascular Health Study, a
longitudinal study sponsored by the National Institutes of Health of more
than 5,000 older adults recruited from four academic medical centers. A
longitudinal study means people sign up to have their health followed over
long periods of time. (The most famous of these types of studies is the
Framingham Heart Study mentioned in Chapter 4.) The research group
found no relationship between caffeine consumption and the numbers
of premature beats from the atria (PACs) or ventricles (PVCs). This non-
relationship persisted after adjustment of possible confounding factors.[2]

Caffeine and AF. The evidence that caffeine does not associate
with AF is even stronger. In 2013, a research team from Portugal culled
together seven studies that included more than 115,000 individuals. They
found that caffeine exposure was not associated with an increased risk of
AF. What's more, when only the highest-quality studies were considered,
the researchers found a 15 percent reduction in AF with low-dose caffeine
exposure.[3] A larger study from a group of Chinese researchers confirmed
these findings, including the same sign of AF protection with low-dose
caffeine exposure.[4]

Caffeine and electrical properties of the heart. Caffeine exposure has
been tested in a randomized clinical trial in patients with known arrhythmia. Canadian researchers studied 80 patients who were to have catheter ablation of supraventricular tachycardia (SVT). One hour before the
procedure, half the group received caffeine tablets, and the other half
received a placebo. Although caffeine increased blood pressure, it did not
have any effects on the measured electrical properties of the heart.[5]

Caffeine and general cardiac health. The largest study on caffeine and heart disease included more than 1.2 million participants. In this case, researchers reviewed 36 studies from the literature and found that moderate coffee consumption (3 to 5 cups per day) associated with a lower risk for heart attack, stroke, or death related to heart disease.[6] Yes, lower.

An important caveat is that most of these studies look at populations, not individuals. That means that although certain people may not be sensitive to caffeine, others—perhaps, you—could be quite sensitive to it.

We know this information sounds counterintuitive. We've heard from many athletes who feel less arrhythmia after reducing or eliminating caffeine intake. The confusing thing about heart rhythm problems is that it's hard to sort out what caused the reduction in symptoms. Heart arrhythmias have natural variability, so it might be mere circumstance. Another possibility is that when people get a diagnosis of a heart problem, they adjust things besides caffeine consumption, such as the amount of training they do or sleep they get, or what they eat. Doctors call these things confounding factors.

The caffeine revelation has caused a significant reversal in thinking. Doctors ask patients with arrhythmia to give up a lot: alcohol, training, stressful situations, and more. It's nice that athletes can enjoy an espresso without guilt.

Preparation for your doctor's visit

Let's say you have decided to see a doctor. You have an appointment. What's the best way to prepare for it? Doctors are usually busy; you want to get the most from your visit. Here are some pointers.

Show up early

At least in the United States, you will have lots of paperwork to complete. Part of this paperwork will include a brief survey of organ systems. There are two reasons your doctor asks you to fill out these questions. One is that your answers to the survey could alert him or her to unusual symptoms. Another, more practical reason, is that your insurance company requires them in order to pay your billing claim.

When you fill out the survey, focus on what's most important and recent. If you check every box in a long list of symptoms, you risk distracting your doctor. By all means, note pertinent and bothersome problems, but don't get hung up on a rash that occurred 10 years ago.

Prepare your history

When you meet the doctor in the exam room, he or she will start with the history, or the story, of your problems. Although the history is the least objective aspect of your visit, it is the most important part of the doctor-patient interaction. One of the most helpful things you can do is to go over your story before your visit. Be organized. Be complete, but be brief.

In the evaluation of a possible cardiac problem, doctors ask first about the big three symptoms: chest pain, breathlessness, and fainting. If you have any of these symptoms, be ready to describe the sensations and the situations that bring them on, or the things that give relief. How often do they occur? What were you doing? Are they predictable—that is, do they occur every time you exert yourself? In the case of fainting, were there warning signs, or did you pass out stone-cold all of a sudden?

Another question, and an important way of sorting out the condition of the heart, is to determine whether you can sometimes perform high-level exertion and sometimes not. Many of the rhythm problems experienced by athletes are intermittent. I always ask my patients, "When your heart is in rhythm, how well do you perform?" If you usually feel strong except for the days or hours when the heart is not in rhythm, it suggests that your heart could be structurally normal.

Another important part of the history is the duration of the symptoms. Have they been occurring for a few days or weeks, or have they been present for years?

A key point that you need to understand is that most doctors are rushed for time. You can help this situation by telling your story efficiently. I've had athletes drone on for many minutes about the minutia of their training. This wastes time. The doctor's eyes will glaze over if you discuss your lactate threshold, VO_2max, or threshold power.

Of course, you want the doctor to understand your athletic lifestyle, but that can be conveyed quickly. An easy way to relay your athleticism to the doctor is to report a typical weekly training burden, in hours or miles of activity per week. You could even say that you are a "serious" athlete, or, for emphasis, a "very serious athlete." Remember, most doctors consider a bike ride of 20–30 minutes to be a lot of exercise. You need to make it clear that your activity level is considerably greater.

Bring useful data

You don't want to underplay your commitment to exercise, but brevity and the relevance of your data are critical. Your doctor probably doesn't use a Garmin. He or she likely has not heard of Strava, and there's almost no chance your doctor understands heart-rate variability indices.

In getting the right diagnosis and treatment, your precise numerical data are far less relevant than your story and physical findings. Keep the data simple. Doctors are not training coaches.

If your resting heart rate is trending up, just say "my resting heart rate is trending up." If you are having difficulty getting to max heart rate, just say so. If you have a recording in which your rate jumps from 140 to 200 bpm during a ride, bring a screenshot and show it. Say, "Look, doc, this is what happens when I feel funny sensations in my chest."

If you keep a calendar of days when your heart is irregular, bring a summary. Doctors want to know if your heart is out of rhythm one day a year or 15 days a month. Whether it's precisely 12 days or 18 days does not matter.

Past medical history, social history, and family history

After the storytelling (doctors call this the "history of present illness") comes your past medical history (PMH), social history (SH), and family history (FH).

In the PMH, the doctor wants to know whether you have other diseases such as diabetes or hypertension or prior surgeries that could be relevant, such as heart procedures. A few things in your SH are important to convey, including tobacco use, alcohol and/or illicit drug use, and your occupation. Both alcohol and drugs play a role in heart disease and heart rhythm problems. It is important to be honest about these questions. Doctors and their staff are bound by strict privacy standards, and there's no reason to hide the more unsavory aspects of your medical history.

Your occupation is important because it gives the doctor a sense of who you are as a person. Specifically, your occupation gives the doctor a sense of the daily stresses that you may experience. Airline pilots, for example, work varying shifts, and shift work is stressful on the heart rhythm. Pastors repeatedly deal with stressful situations in their parish. They travel often and spend lots of time helping others. That means they may have less time for their own health. Engineers are usually detail oriented. They like to understand why and how the heart jumped out of rhythm. (If only it were that easy to know.)

FH focuses on cardiac issues. It's relevant if one of your first-degree relatives suffered premature (before age 60) sudden cardiac death or premature heart disease. If your parents are alive after age 75, you likely have good genes. The doctor doesn't need to know your elderly parents' medical problems.

Physical exam

After the history-taking comes the physical exam. An often overlooked but important exam finding are the three vital signs of blood pressure, heart rate, and respiratory rate. These may have been taken by the nurse or medical assistant.

The doctor's part of the exam will include inspection (yes, he will look at you and notice things—probably your athletic body shape, or lack thereof), palpation, and auscultation with a stethoscope. A skilled physician can obtain a lot of information from a careful exam. It's certain that the doctor will listen carefully to your heart. During this part of the exam, it may not seem like the doctor is doing much, but the presence of abnormal sounds, such as a heart murmur or irregular rhythm, might suggest further testing.

Electrocardiogram

The final part of the information gathering during an office visit is the 12-lead electrocardiogram (ECG). The easiest way to understand the ECG is to think of each of the electrical leads as different viewfinders to your heart's electrical system. The right arm's lead looks at the heart's activation from the right and the left arm's lead from the left. The leg leads look up at the heart, while the chest leads look from front to back. The pattern of the electrical activation of the heart provides an immense amount of information. An ECG is sort of like a fingerprint.

Some parts of the ECG are objective, but others are more subjective. Let's first take the objective aspects of the ECG, and then we can get into the trickier parts where pattern recognition plays a role.

If we assume a good-quality recording (which can be achieved if the technician makes sure there is no movement and all the electrodes have good skin contact), an ECG is quite accurate at recording time intervals. The time it takes the electrical impulse to go from north (atria) to south (ventricle) is called the PR interval (P refers to the atria and R to ventricles). The time it takes the heart to contract is called the QRS duration, and the time it takes the heart to relax is the QT interval (see Figure 5.2).

You may have heard the term "QT interval." It's an important measure because prolongation of this interval can lead to sudden death from

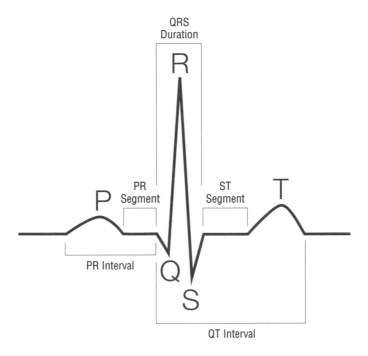

FIGURE 5.2. An ECG trace of one cardiac cycle

ventricular arrhythmia. The relaxation time of the heart can be prolonged by congenital diseases or by "acquired causes" such as prescription or nonprescription drugs. Other causes include severe electrolyte depletion, particularly potassium, and magnesium deficiency. The good news is that if the QT interval is normal, the odds are that you don't have Long QT syndrome (a condition that can cause rapid, chaotic heartbeats and may lead to fainting or seizures).

Now to the trickier parts of the ECG. There are normal patterns and abnormal patterns. And then there are "nonspecific" patterns, meaning they could be either normal or abnormal.

Athletes pose a challenge to ECG readers. Endurance training causes the heart to adapt. These changes, most of which are normal—even desired—can cause ECG patterns that can confuse doctors.

A little further on, we will talk more about the fact that most doctors don't grasp the mental, emotional, and physical demands placed on the endurance athlete. As for ECG testing, a group of expert sports cardiologists have put together athlete-specific guidelines called the "Seattle Criteria" to aid in the use of ECG for athletes. It's beyond the scope of this book to go into the details, but the gist is that they expand the "normal" patterns to include those typically seen in athletes. A brief example is that the Seattle Criteria allow for a normal heart rate to be as low as 30 beats per minute.[7]

History, exam, and ECG: These are the basic components of the initial medical assessment. They give your doctor a good idea of the presence or absence of structural heart disease (scary or not scary). Sometimes it isn't clear. Two other basic medical tests your doctor may order are the echocardiogram and treadmill exercise stress test.

Echocardiogram

An "echo," as it is called, is an ultrasound of the heart. In much the same way that an ECG takes a multiple electrical view of the heart, an echo takes multiple (five to six) ultrasound slices of the heart. A technician uses a probe to see the heart from a variety of angles.

An echo can measure the size of the heart's four chambers, the strength of right and left ventricular muscle contraction known as the ejection fraction (the percentage of blood leaving your heart each time it contracts), the function of the four heart valves, and the condition of some of the surrounding structures.

Doctors love the echo because it delivers lots of information without any pain or radiation. It's a great tool for ruling out dangerous heart conditions. Earlier we noted that most athletes don't have structural heart disease. But some do; an echo can often diagnose these conditions. Three examples of diseases an echo can see immediately include

- Hypertrophic cardiomyopathy: This is an abnormal thickening of the heart muscle, usually of the septum between the right and left ventricle. It's an important disease to know about because it can lead to sudden death due to arrhythmia in the ventricle.

- Cardiomyopathy: This is a medical term describing disease of the heart muscle. It can affect either the right or left ventricle. An echo sees this as poorly contracting or contracting segments of the ventricle. Similar to hypertrophic cardiomyopathy, cardiomyopathy can also lead to sudden death from arrhythmia in the ventricle.

- Valvular heart disease: This is a broad category of disease that affects one or more of the four heart valves. Heart valves can either be stenotic (too tight) or regurgitant (too leaky). The echo assesses the valves either by direct sight or with Doppler (like weather Doppler). An important caveat about echo assessment of valves is that the Doppler is very sensitive. Many normal people have mild degrees of regurgitation. Don't be alarmed if you have seen a report that says you have "mild" valve regurgitation.

The purpose of going through these three possible echo findings is that if you have a normal echo, you should feel relieved that you don't have any of the most common causes of serious structural heart disease.

There is still one more possibility that a doctor will consider, one that an exam, ECG, and echo may not see. That is the possibility of blockages in the coronary arteries. As you recall from Chapter 1, the blood vessels on the outside of the heart are the ones that deliver nutrients to the beating heart.

Exercise stress test

The exercise stress test is an extremely useful tool, especially for an athlete who may have symptoms during exertion. The test is simple: The doctor records an ECG first while you are at rest and then again while you work through increasing degrees of exercise. Exercise places an increased demand on the heart, so the test reveals how well the heart responds. Will it be able to deliver the added blood supply to meet the demand? How will the heart rhythm behave during stress?

If there are serious blockages in the coronary arteries, the ECG will show strain patterns when demand outstrips supply during the test. That's called a "positive" stress test.

In addition to looking for blockages, two other findings of a stress test provide useful information. The first of these is exercise tolerance.

Simply stated, this is the time one can exercise on a standard protocol of increasing workloads, usually on a treadmill. Many studies have correlated the duration of exercise as a strong predictor of future cardiac events. In nonathletes, we shoot for greater than 10 minutes of walking on a standard protocol. That doesn't seem like much to an endurance athlete, but it is highly predictive of a good future prognosis.

The second valuable piece of data doctors get from an exercise stress test is the presence or absence of rhythm problems. This test doesn't always provoke an arrhythmia, but when it does, it's reassuring, because now we have the right diagnosis.

These are the basics. Doctors listen to your story and your past history. They examine your body. They study your ECG and possibly look at the heart via ultrasound and/or assess your heart's response to stress. None of these tests involve any needles in the body or exposure to radiation. Doctors call them "noninvasive" evaluations. This cascade of evaluation serves the dual purpose of determining risk (whether you have something scary or not scary) and the search for a diagnosis.

The doctor's blindness to the endurance athlete

One of the drawbacks you may face in your exam is the fact that most doctors have little experience with a full-fledged endurance athlete. If you have trained for hours on hours, months on months, years on years, or if you compete in races, you are special. Your heart and body and mind have undergone adaptations that most doctors don't regularly see.

We mentioned training-related adaptations when it came to ECG patterns, but athletes present more than just variable patterns on an electrical record of the heart. A competitive endurance athlete lives a different kind of life than most people who seek out the services of a doctor. At least in most Western countries, the vast majority of people who go to the doctor have diseases acquired from too little exercise, not too much.

Here is an outlandish example of what I mean: One of my colleagues, an experienced private-practice cardiologist, once remarked to me, "John, it's not as if riding a bike is that hard. My gosh, it's not like weight lifting or football or hockey." He was serious. His view of bike riding was that of the beach cruiser: When you are tired, you slow down.

Most doctors don't know the sensation of being in a road race, criterium, or time trial. They've never been in the gutter because of a crosswind, saying to themselves, *Ten more pedal strokes, just do it for 10 more pedal strokes. Hold that wheel! Don't let go!*

Most doctors don't know the effort it takes to bridge across to a breakaway. When normal people feel the sensation that a curtain is closing in on their peripheral vision, they turn the tension down on the exercise bike or reduce the speed of the treadmill. They pull the plug on the pain. They are normal. Competitive athletes are not.

Even doctors who run marathons don't quite get the intensity thing. Marathons are a different sort of affair. There is no question that they are hard, but they generally have an even pace and don't involve the competitive crises that flare up repeatedly in a bicycle race or a cross-country ski race or a triathlon.

But it isn't just the intensity of the efforts that most doctors don't get; the demands of training remain unfathomable. When normal people are tired or sick or busy with life, they don't go ride or run for hours. Exercise for normal people is expendable. Yes, it is true that many normal people exercise on a schedule, but they typically walk, jog, or do yoga.

Here is the key difference between "normal" exercise and training. In normal exercise, it's clear that when one is finished with the activity, it gave more life force than it took away. Tell me that's the case after a four-hour training ride in intense heat. It's not. Most doctors don't know that training can break people down. They think exercise builds people up. If you are an athlete, or live with one, you know differently.

Another aspect of the training life that most doctors don't get is the mental aspect. That you would worry about missing a breakaway in next weekend's criterium—worry about it on a Monday!—is utterly foreign. They see you as a professional with a job, wife, and family, but they do not get your focus on increasing threshold power by 10 watts in the next month. Little do they know the means you will take to get to those ends.

These gaps in knowledge set the stage for both overdiagnosis and underdiagnosis. Let's talk first about overdiagnosis. As we described in Chapter 2, prolonged and intense training induces adaptations in the heart. The heart is a muscle. It will grow larger, thicker, and stronger with exercise. As the volume of blood pumped (stroke volume) increases with training, heart rate will drop.

Low heart rate may be the most common overdiagnosis made in athletes. When doctors were medical students, they learned the normal resting heart rate ranged between 55 and 100 beats per minute. That is true but incomplete. The resting heart rate follows a distribution first described by Professor Carl Friedrich Gauss in the 18th century. You may know the Gaussian distribution as a normal bell curve. Most people, in fact, do have resting heart rates between 55 and 100 bpm, but there are normal people on the tails of the curve. Athletes, most commonly, live on the low end of resting heart rates.

I was once at a European heart meeting where a doctor presented a case including an ECG that showed a heart rate of 32 beats per minute. The presenter withheld the fact that the ECG belonged to an athlete. He then asked the audience which treatment they would recommend. The audience response system, an automated way to ask the audience questions and compile the most common answers, revealed that a significant number of attendees recommended a pacemaker.

Before the first presenter could clarify things, a fiery senior presenter stepped to the microphone and chastised the audience. He was visibly angry. He used the example of five-time Tour de France champion Miguel Indurain, who famously boasted a resting heart rate of 28 bpm. I can't claim definite knowledge of the great Spanish champion's heart rate, but I routinely see athletes from high to low caliber with heart rates in this range.

The key to understanding a low heart rate is simple: symptoms. If the heart rate is 30 and the patient feels well, then there are no worries. If, however, the heart rate is 30 and the patient is fainting or breathless, that is a different matter. (There's also a difference between a low heart rate due to the normal sinus [north to south] rhythm and a low heart rate due to a complete AV block [south to north] pattern. The former is benign; the latter is rarely benign.)

If heart rate is the most commonly misunderstood athletic finding, enlargement of the heart is the next most common. One of the defining debates in the field of sports cardiology comes in deciding when an enlarged and thickened heart is due to normal adaptation and when it's due to hypertrophic cardiomyopathy. It's a huge issue; on one side of the line lies perfect health, and on the other lurks a life-threatening disease.

Sorting out the athletic heart from a diseased heart demonstrates the inexperience of most doctors with the athletic condition. Even the well-trained, experienced adult cardiologist is not accustomed to seeing the patterns of a thin-chest-walled trained athlete. The thin chest wall can come into play because the ECG records voltage, and when the ECG's electrical wires are closer to the heart, they see bigger signals. Bigger signals on an ECG can fool doctors into thinking the heart is enlarged.

In addition, when it comes to echocardiography, the athlete lying supine in a bed will have very low levels of adrenaline. That can make the strength of the heart contraction look weaker, even though it's not.

It's beyond the scope of this book to list every possible confusing abnormality that athletes bring to the medical evaluation; suffice it to say, there are many. We don't mean to imply that most or even many diagnoses made in athletes are wrong. Instead, it's important for you to know that scant few diagnoses are certain. The problem is that doctors don't like to miss things—especially in athletes, who will push themselves to extraordinary limits. This is why overdiagnosis is common in athletes. Think of it from the doctor's perspective—they feel there's more danger from underdiagnosis than overdiagnosis.

It is, therefore, a good idea to respectfully ask the doctor what his or her level of certainty is. I love it when patients ask me this. Good doctors rarely object. Good doctors understand that every call they make has a level of certainty. I often respond to requests to diagnose a pattern on an ECG with both the answer and my level of certainty.

Overdiagnosis may not seem like a problem to you. You might think, "Better safe than sorry; let's be complete, do all the tests." But in the real world, medical tests are not perfect—especially in athletes.

I've seen overtesting cause severe harm. Take the case of a 45-year-old doctor who complained of funny sensations in his chest. A monitor showed simple PACs, which led to an echocardiogram and stress test. He had an athletic heart and nonspecific findings on the stress test, even though he nearly set a record for time staying on the treadmill. Given these "fuzzy" findings, the doctor thought it best to do an invasive test called a heart catheterization.

"Cath," as it is called in the medical world, is a test in which a doctor inserts a catheter into each of the coronary arteries, and then injects contrast dye down the vessel to look for blockages. The complication rate for the 20-minute test is very low, but not zero. Unfortunately, this high-performing patient with benign skipped beats suffered a major heart attack when the plastic catheter injured his coronary artery (in medical terminology, "dissected" it). He survived but suffered damage to his heart.

This case illustrates the problem of doing too many tests. Each test has a chance of delivering a "false positive," and each invasive test has a small risk of complications.

Underdiagnosis, which means there was a problem but the doctor missed it, is less common for athletes. It is uncommon because, at least in the United States, doctors have a low threshold for ordering tests and a high threshold for calling the results normal. In fact, some doctors feel "normal" is one of the toughest calls in medicine.

One of the worst cases of underdiagnosis I've seen was a middle-aged marathon runner who kept complaining of wheezing while running. He diagnosed himself with asthma, and his impression helped convince his doctor it was asthma. But increasing doses of asthma inhalers did not help him. The breathing worsened.

One day he passed out while running. When the paramedics arrived, it was evident he was having a heart attack. All this time, a worsening blockage in one of his coronary arteries was slowly closing off. Fortunately, he underwent surgery and did well.

Why were the patient and doctor so easily fooled? Hindsight is always sharp, but one of the reasons is the misconception that athleticism and fitness inoculate one from getting regular (atherosclerotic) heart disease. As we discussed in Chapter 4, exercise and cardio-respiratory fitness reduce the risk of heart disease, but that risk is not eliminated.

The moral of this story is to beware of anchoring bias. Both the patient and doctor were anchored to the idea that asthma was causing the breathing problem. The key to preventing underdiagnosis is to pay attention to symptoms that do not relent despite treatment. But be warned; overdiagnosis is much more common.

What's stopping you from seeking medical attention?

The best person to answer the question of why you haven't sought medical help for symptoms is you. Here are some key questions:

- Is your well-honed ability to push through pain masking symptoms of real disease?

- Are your symptoms something you can correct with rest?

- Have you tried decreasing your training load, reducing alcohol intake, or eating better?

I've seen athletes push through severe symptoms of disease. It's remarkable what an athlete can ignore. It's impossible to quantify one's pain threshold, but heart disease can come on slowly. The stealthy creep of heart disease can blend with stoicism to mask important symptoms. Be mindful of this. It's real.

Recently, a group of researchers assessed symptoms in the month before a cardiac arrest in more than 800 patients older than the age of 50.[8] The research team found that half the group had warning symptoms— mostly chest pain or shortness of breath. Although the study authors acknowledge the potential for recall bias (surviving patients may be looking for an explanation), these results underscore the need to pay attention to warning symptoms.

I've seen athletes who were clearly overtrained, overstressed, or some combination thereof. My background as a doctor as well as a patient with exercise-induced atrial fibrillation helps me sort out the difference between real disease and being overcooked. But this is a challenging situation. It's not always so easy. Many doctors will struggle with that history. They don't always know the right questions to ask an athlete.

If you take nothing else away from this chapter, remember these three messages. First, ignoring clear symptoms like chest pain, fainting, or breathlessness is unwise. Second, many symptoms may respond to simple measures, such as rest or attention to diet and removal of cardiac irritants. And third, when you seek medical attention, be prepared to help your doctor make the right diagnosis with the minimum of testing.

CASE STUDY
Genevieve Halvorsen: Atrial flutter, atrial fibrillation
First episode at 41

CHRIS CASE

Genevieve Halvorsen started cycling at the age of 13. She competed in her first race at 14. (Before that she was a competitive swimmer.) She competed into young adulthood and then dialed it back when she became pregnant. In her early 40s, she joined a women's cycling group in the San Francisco area and began training for centuries (100-mile rides) in and around the hills of the Bay Area. How did she feel about cycling? In a word, fanatical. It dovetailed with her competitive personality.

In 1998, at the age of 41, she noticed some weakness when she rode. She thought she wasn't training enough. She let it go for a while. But when she started waking up with severe palpitations, a racing heart, in a sweat, she knew something serious was upon her.

It would take 10 years for doctors to find the correct diagnosis.

She was first told she had an anxiety disorder and was prescribed antidepressants.

"I have an athletic build. I'm pretty young looking, so when I went to the doctor, they're not thinking A-fib like they would for a 75-year-old obese guy," she says. "I did not fit any doctor's idea of a heart patient."

She felt slow on the bike when she was taking antidepressants. She'd think, "I've got to ride even more!" At that point she didn't ride with a heart rate monitor. She'd never heard of arrhythmias, and she certainly didn't know anyone with one, so she trusted what she was told. "The doctor must be right, I thought. I must be anxious."

In 2007, her episodes became more severe. She underwent a stress test, though her doctor, unfamiliar with the physiological characteristics of endurance athletes, only had her raise her heart rate to 150 beats per minute on a treadmill before ending the test. "Get out of here, there's nothing wrong with your heart," he told her. "You're having panic attacks."

Her symptoms remained paroxysmal: sudden, short, frequent recurrences or intensifications of tachycardia.

In April 2008, while commuting to work by bike, she experienced such a severe and scary episode—her elevated heart rate would not subside no matter what she did—that she headed to urgent care. She was given a Holter monitor, a portable device that records the rhythm of the heart continuously (typically for 24 to 48 hours) via electrodes attached to the chest.

She went out for a ride the next day. "Less than two miles into the ride, bang! Arrhythmia." Ten years after her initial scare, she was finally diagnosed with right atrial flutter and AF.

"When I was first diagnosed, I rode up into the hills by myself and cried," Halvorsen says. "I thought, 'I am never going to be able to do this again.' Cycling was such a big part of me. Being with my friends on bikes is a really big part of my identity. The doctors were like, 'Well, you're still walking around and you're still alive. What's the big deal?' I was always worried a doctor was just going to say, 'Well, just don't ride like that anymore.'"

Why did it take so long for Halvorsen to be correctly diagnosed? In her mind, being female played a significant role. As she sought answers to her heart issues, she had a series of young female primary care physicians. One even wrote in her chart, "Has magical and mythical thinking about her heart. Has a generalized anxiety disorder." Halvorsen discovered this stupefying diagnosis after asking for her medical charts as she transitioned from one doctor to another in her quest.

"Maybe you don't find as many female A-fib patients because doctors think all women are just anxious," she laughs. "Actually, it happens a lot. I've seen on forums and on Facebook where people have written that the doctor thinks they had an anxiety disorder."

After a decade of searching, she could finally seek treatment for her arrhythmia. She immediately began reading up on ablations. Her husband, an avid runner, had heard of many long-distance runners who were turning to ablation for treatment. She quickly decided this was what she wanted.

She had been prescribed a number of different medications over the course of the many years it took for her to be correctly diagnosed, including beta-blockers. "Anyone who has ever been on them will tell you as soon as you go up any kind of hill, you are out of breath," Halvorsen says. "The idea of being on some kind of pill for my whole life, it was like, 'Wow, ablation works?' At that point, they were like, with ablation you'll be cured. That's when I said give it to me."

Her first ablation was performed in 2008. She was back to exercising two weeks later. Unfortunately, she never felt the same afterward, and after seven months she was back where she started.

She was prescribed a series of anti-arrhythmic drugs and found support through online forums. That's also where she learned of Dr. Andrea Natale, whom she describes as "the best" electrophysiologist in the world. He eventually performed her second ablation in 2010. While Dr. Natale considered his procedure to be the first true ablation, he also reasoned she might eventually have to have a third due to the delicate nature of the area in which it was located. "He didn't want to overdo it all at once," Halvorsen says.

The prediction was right. Halvorsen developed a pattern of heart rate jumps: If she stopped during a ride, for example, her heart rate would fall to 110 beats per minute and then suddenly shoot up to about 200. It turned out to be an atrial flutter, which she says could have been caused by the second ablation. So, in 2011, she underwent a third ablation to treat a left atrial flutter.

At first, soon after this third procedure, she would push up against the limits of what she thought was possible with her newly ablated heart. She'd ride hard, trying to seek that invisible limit.

Now, three and a half years later, at the age of 58, she questions whether she wants to put herself through another ablation procedure. "I would do it again, if it got bad. I would, if they would let me do it," she says.

But, she admits, she doesn't ride as much anymore. Or as far. She still rides with her cycling group, but she stays away from big hills. "I constantly worry that I'm going to put myself back into A-fib." She wears her heart rate monitor religiously, even on commutes. And she wonders why it happened to her.

"I feel very strongly it was caused by all the riding and training I did over the years," she says. "I've read the studies that say given the training amount and the number of years I did it, it wouldn't be unusual to develop an arrhythmia. And if you think about me riding intensely starting at age 14 . . .

"I'm also always dehydrated," she continues. "The combination of long-term endurance training and chronic electrolyte imbalance makes you think, 'Yeah, that's gonna happen.'"

It is worth viewing Halvorsen's case history in the broader context of women's medical diagnoses. Research on cardiac misdiagnoses reported in the *New England Journal of Medicine,* for example, looked at more than 10,000 heart patients (48 percent of them women) who had gone to their hospital emergency rooms with chest pain or other significant heart attack symptoms.[9] Women younger than 55 were seven times more likely to be misdiagnosed and turned away from the ER than their male counterparts. It would seem that in terms of the delay of an accurate diagnosis, there is strong evidence that being female was a contributing factor.

In 2008, a Cornell University study titled "Gender Bias in the Diagnosis, Treatment, and Interpretation of Coronary Heart Disease Symptoms" examined whether physicians tend to evaluate heart patients differently despite comparable symptoms and risk factors, based solely on their gender.[10]

Half of the patient charts used in this study indicated that a patient had recently experienced a significant life stressor and that they appeared anxious. Each physician read one version of the record and was then asked to specify a diagnosis, make treatment recommendations, and indicate the probable cause of the described symptoms.

Results showed a significant gender bias when heart disease symptoms were presented in the context of stress, with fewer women receiving coronary heart disease diagnoses (15 percent versus 56 percent), cardiologist referrals (30 percent versus 62 percent), and prescriptions of cardiac medication (13 percent versus 47 percent) compared to the men.

Researchers also found that the presence of stress shifted the interpretation of women's chest pain, shortness of breath, and irregular heart rate so that these were thought to have a psychological origin.

By contrast, men's symptoms were perceived as cardiac whether or not emotional stressors were present.

6 | Getting the news

LENNARD ZINN

ONE DAY YOU'RE OUT riding, skiing, running, walking, swimming, paddling, rowing. Or you're just standing, sitting, or lying around, and you feel something strange in your chest. What do you do?

You're a lifelong athlete, and you've always had a great heart that got you through many hard races and training sessions, always delivering the blood your muscles and brain needed. (Admittedly, there may have been times you wished that it would have given you just a bit more oxygen-rich blood when you were suffering mightily, trying to keep up in the race or maintain the pace in training. But still . . .) At rest, it beats at a nice, strong, steady rate. Your low heartbeat impresses friends and nurses, as does your low blood pressure. What could go wrong? After all, you lead a superhealthy life. You get lots of exercise and are generally outside in the fresh air for a couple of hours every day. You watch what you eat and drink, you don't smoke, and you're lean and fit.

Perhaps you have felt an occasional skipped heartbeat while you're sitting or lying around, and perhaps you've been told by experts that it's nothing to worry about. They may have even given it a name or an acronym, like PAC (for premature atrial complex). So you may have some experience with your heart not always being in perfect rhythm, but it always rose to the occasion in racing and training.

You certainly don't want to believe there is anything wrong with your heart. More to the point, deep down, although you perhaps can't see it at the time, you don't want to know. Even if something is wrong, much of your identity is based on being fit and fast and an amazement to your not-so-fit friends and acquaintances, especially ones of a similar age. A heart condition doesn't work with that image.

You also don't want any pity or concern from people, especially ones whom you could always outdo if it ever came to a competition. Furthermore, much of your social life is built around training and racing with your buddies, and you don't want to give that up.

You do plan to live a lot longer, however, and feeling weird stuff in your heart carries with it some unease. Do you go to the doctor? Or do you ignore it, figuring it will just go away?

If you use a heart rate monitor when training or racing, and you felt something odd while doing so—felt your heart rate spike, or flutter, or skip a beat—you might have some unequivocal evidence one way or the other. Download it and look at it carefully. If you saw that same spike on a heart rate graph of a good friend, your spouse, or your child, would you tell them to go see a doctor about it? If the answer is yes, then go.

If the odd feeling didn't happen while exercising, you won't have any heart monitor data. But the AliveCor Kardia ECG smartphone app is perfect for that circumstance. You put the AliveCor unit on the back of or adjacent to a smartphone or tablet computer on which you've downloaded the app. Sit down, relax, open the Kardia app, select "Record now," and place your fingertips on the two large, square, metal electrodes and gently keep them there. It will record for 30 seconds, drawing an ever-smoother graph as the seconds pass, after which it will read out something like "Normal," "Unclassified," or "Unreadable" or perhaps will indicate an arrhythmia like AF. Obviously, if it reads that your heart is in arrhythmia, go see a doctor. If it reads Unclassified or Unreadable, keep trying. Relax. Don't squeeze the electrodes so hard.

If you have no electronic data to inform you one way or the other, base your decision about whether to see a specialist on the "Warning symptoms" section in Chapter 5.

Finding the right doctor

If you haven't ended up in the emergency room with this problem, you will have some choice about the first doctor you go to. Even if you went in with this issue via the ER and then perhaps even wound your way through the cardio test lab and/or a hospital stay, you still will have some choice about the doctor(s) you see in the future. And if you decide to have surgical intervention, it makes sense to see a few doctors before settling on the one to work with.

As you learned in Chapter 5, many doctors do not get much exposure to the particular electrical problems of athletes. Whether there is a doctor near you with such experience can certainly be a function of where you live. If you live in an active community teeming with masters athletes, you might not be much of an exception in a cardiology practice there. When I went to see a cardiac electrophysiologist at a huge teaching hospital in Denver, the cardiac risk factors of the people in the waiting room were plain to see. There were people outside smoking, and inside were people who were overweight, in wheelchairs, and/or hooked up to oxygen. However, in the waiting room of my electrophysiologist in Boulder, I rarely see people that are obviously heart patients, and there are almost always fit-looking people waiting.

The best way to start your search for a doctor is to get recommendations for cardiologists from other athletes whom you trust who have experienced heart problems. It may be that your insurance requires you to first go to your primary care physician, who then will refer you to a specialist. In that case, if you can't go to the cardiologist(s) others recommended to you, get a referral to one your doctor recommends.

Cardiologists are roughly split between plumbers and electricians, and if you know that your problem is not with your plumbing (a category that for our purposes would include congenital heart problems, valve problems, and so on), then that narrows it down to electrophysiologists. Some doctors you will relate to, and some you won't, so seek out one whom you feel comfortable talking to and who answers your questions clearly. Be willing to switch to a different doctor if you don't click with the first one. And, if you are going to have an ablation performed, you should be aware that some electrophysiologists are particularly skilled in ablating some types of arrhythmias and are perhaps not so effective with other types. So get as many recommendations as you can from people whom you trust who are also knowledgeable about your particular diagnosis.

As Dr. Mandrola mentioned in Chapter 5, the doctor doesn't need to know your whole athletic history, what races you have coming up, and where you think you'll place in them. However, I have found that cardiologists often appreciate seeing printouts of heart rate graphs downloaded from a heart rate monitor that show where the heart spiked up or down. Write down the questions that you especially want the doctor to answer so that you don't leave his or her office slapping your forehead, having forgotten to ask something important. Bring someone along to take notes, as you may find that the information you're receiving is so confounding, scary, new, or unintelligible that you can't take it all in at the time or remember it later. Review what you've learned immediately afterward.

Tests, tests, and more tests

As soon as you walk into a cardiologist's office, expect to have a technician hook you up to an electrocardiograph (ECG) machine. Apart from that basic test, you have the ultimate say about whether you'll perform a particular test or not, and you might have an indication of whether it will be useful or not.

For example, a cardiac stress test on a treadmill or perhaps on a stationary bicycle is common. The patient is hooked up via wires and electrodes to an ECG machine and must periodically increase his or her power, either due to the treadmill becoming steeper and moving faster, or due to increased resistance of the stationary bike while maintaining a constant pedaling cadence. For most people, this is the hardest physical exercise they'll do all month or all year. But for you, it may be easier than many interval workouts you do regularly. If you know that your heart doesn't ever do anything strange in similar or more intense interval workouts, then perhaps it doesn't make sense to fork over whatever the cardiac stress test costs (I have been charged over $2,100 for each of my treadmill stress tests). This is particularly true if you know that you have no plumbing problems, as you may have confirmed if you've had an angiogram (also known as catheterization).

If your doctor feels that a particular test would be useful for you to perform, however, take that advice. The whole point of searching for doctors you trust and have rapport with is to believe them when they tell you what they think will be good for you.

Stages of denial, and what it may take to get the message

For someone who is habituated to being fit and competitive in racing endurance events, getting the news that your heart may not allow you to do what you've become accustomed to doing will not go down easily. It is completely natural to go into denial for a while. I don't know of any masters athletes diagnosed with non-life-threatening arrhythmias who didn't go back to pushing it hard in training or racing in hopes that the incident that sent them to a cardiologist was just a fluke.

In my case, when I went to the emergency room on my primary care physician's insistence, the ER doc on duty was none other than Shannon Sovndal, a team doctor for the Garmin-Sharp pro cycling team. Had he not had such stellar credentials with top athletes, I might have dismissed his findings of elevated troponin in my bloodstream and his consequent instruction for me to transfer (via ambulance!) to the main cardiac unit downtown, where I would spend the night and be in the lab the next morning with catheters threaded into my arteries.

Once convinced that I had truly experienced a significant arrhythmic event, I came up with many theories for what might have brought it on, and I tested each one. For instance, I decided that I must have been low on electrolytes when it happened, so I stopped drinking plain water while riding and skiing and switched to an electrolyte mix instead. That seemed to work for a while; I got in some hard workouts with no problems, but the atrial tachycardia eventually returned.

After electrolyte replacement failed to eliminate my arrhythmia, I decided that I must have been too stressed and not getting a sufficient warm up before hard efforts, so I stopped driving to cyclocross races and only raced the ones I could ride to. I'd get to races with a nice, relaxing warm-up, without any frantic loading and unloading of the car with spare bikes and wheels. That worked for a while, in part because it limited the total number of races I did, which stressed my heart less. But then the arrhythmia reared up again anyway, and I finally had to admit that it made it impossible to train and race the way I had before.

When even cyclocross racing with a good warm-up and minimal stress resulted in occurrences of arrhythmia, I thought that I could get away with racing less intense events than cyclocross. I tried a long-distance mass-start citizen's gran fondo in Beverly Hills and started slowly, keeping my heart rate below 145 beats per minute. But deep into the race while adhering to my sub-145 rule, tachycardia happened again, and again, and again, until I could only go up the climbs at a crawl without incurring it.

In the end, I believe that all that denial and continued racing and training hard with the hope of retaining some portion of my former life either damaged my heart or trained it so that it now goes into arrhythmia more easily. In the first few months after my first arrhythmia, I could regularly go up to 150 beats per minute without triggering the arrhythmia, but after another six months of training and racing, it would happen at 135 beats per minute and sometimes even well below that. Now I respect that 135 beats per minute limit, and it's (thankfully) held steady there for a couple of years. And after the attempt at ablation on my heart failed, and I was told I'm not a candidate for drug therapies, I just keep my workouts calm and relatively short.

It's not only athletes with non-life-threatening arrhythmias who go through a period of denying their condition. A ski buddy who does have a life-threatening arrhythmia, ventricular tachycardia (V-tach), still tried to ride or ski hard while on beta-blockers. By trying to reclaim some of the old lifestyle he had lost, he was playing Russian roulette, risking another sudden cardiac death (SCD). It wasn't an idle concern, as he has been rescued from SCD with an electric shock numerous times and developed PTSD from it. He doesn't push the limits anymore.

Winston Churchill's quote comes to mind, "You can always count on Americans to do the right thing—after they've tried everything else."

Some people, at least in the short term, may not need to change their lifestyle if they can get a successful cardiac ablation on their first attempt that completely eliminates their symptoms. Many of these people go back to racing at a highly competitive level. If they're happy and doing what they want to do, who am I to say whether moderating their activity level might make more sense in the long run?

One caution about ablation is that its application depends on the arrhythmia. Not all conditions respond to it; difficulties associated with ablating AF, for instance, are detailed in Chapter 8. We've spent a lot of time in this book speaking about heart problems that are (likely) acquired from endurance exercise. Athletes, however, like regular people, can have fluky arrhythmias, such as paroxysmal supraventricular tachycardia (PSVT) or Wolff-Parkinson-White (WPW) syndrome. These rapid heartbeats are due to a congenital aberrant pathway. They can be cured with a catheter ablation procedure, and after a period of recovery, the person can return to the training life because the training life did not cause the problem. Whether or not to change your lifestyle after a successful ablation is a decision that should be based on the type of condition you have (or had), research on the likelihood of recurrence post-ablation under hard training, and advice from doctors whom you trust.

Life after arrhythmia

Just as cardiac arrhythmias cover a wide spectrum of types and symptoms, so does the accommodation to them. What an arrhythmia-prone person can do covers the gamut from having no restrictions (after a successful ablation, for instance) to something close to house arrest for severe cases. And how people respond to any heart-related restrictions also varies widely.

I find that my life is as rich as it was before my first incident of AT, and in many ways it is richer. No, I cannot compete (I could partake, but

I could not be competitive) in bike races and cross-country ski races, and I cannot train as I did before. I also cannot do long-distance, all-day bike rides over multiple high mountain passes. I miss those things greatly, not only the way my body felt and the emotional highs I attained, but also the camaraderie I felt with all the friends who did those things with me.

The other side of that coin is that I now have more freedom to do many other things. Racing takes a lot of time. There are the races themselves, then there's the travel, the equipment preparation, the pre-race and post-race routine. And the training includes not only all the training hours, but also—particularly in the case of something like skiing that most people cannot do right out of their front door—the time spent on transportation back and forth from training venues, as well as on equipment preparation and maintenance, and on constantly loading and unloading equipment in vehicles. I'd guess that by no longer doing ski races and bike races, I have, on average throughout the year, an extra 20 to 40 hours per week to do with as I see fit. That's a lot of time.

While I do still ride my bike and cross-country ski a lot more than the average Joe, I don't do either one every day and don't feel compelled to condition my body for some upcoming event. I enjoy a much broader variety of pursuits now.

I have gone back to doing a lot of things I used to do as a kid, things I had mostly curtailed in the single-minded pursuit of cycling and cross-country skiing. I once again downhill ski, hike, and whitewater kayak (sports I pursued avidly through high school and college) an order of magnitude or two more than I had for many decades. I'm also immensely enjoying newer sports for me, like backcountry skiing and sea kayaking, and I especially appreciate that I have fun doing them during the height of the cyclocross or cross-country-ski seasons, without feeling the slightest pang that I should instead be training for coming races. I continue my twice-weekly full-body sessions with a trainer, and I welcome family and friends to join me in those workouts. All these sports have a social aspect, so I'm enjoying new and old friends in new settings.

I also use some of my extra time and my freedom from preparing for racing to do other leisure activities. I had never had an interest in gardening before, and now I find it to be quite satisfying. Similarly, I never had much interest in fish, but my wife had a koi pond put in right outside my office window with a loud, gushing waterfall I can listen to while working. I enjoy watching and playing with the fish as well as maintaining the pond. When it's 90 degrees outside, now that I am no longer obsessing about missing a bike ride, how can I complain about standing waist-deep in cool water, cleaning filters and pulling out muck, while fish brush against my legs?

I can now travel without bringing a bike or skis with me, and during those trips there is no longer any conversation with my wife and/or daughters about when I'm going to get in my training each day. I find this to be quite freeing, and I think it has deepened my relationships with my family. So has just generally being more available for them when they want me to do something for them; I'm around more, and I don't tend to have an agenda that would preclude me from doing what they ask. I think I was a good husband and father before, but I think I'm better at those things now, and I have a heart arrhythmia to thank for it.

CASE STUDY
Mark Taylor: Undiagnosed
Aged 56

CHRIS CASE

MARK TAYLOR has been feeling strange sensations in his chest intermittently for the past three or four years. His heart rate will rise considerably higher than it used to under similar circumstances and stay elevated for longer. Yet he's never been to a cardiologist. "I don't think I've had anything super-dramatic happen, except unusual feelings. What I feel like I've done is just backed off and stopped pushing it that hard," he says. Taylor's symptoms began not long after the birth of his child, a time when he was sleeping a lot less but still attempting to train hard and balance his career.

During routine physical exams, his general practitioners proclaim him to be fine, nothing to worry about. Sound familiar? If you're like Taylor, you may have dismissed "strange sensations" of your own. Though it's crossed his mind that he should see a cardiologist, Taylor continues to gather information, seeking his own answers.

"When you're in your mid-50s, what am I supposed to be comparing it to?" he asks. "I keep hearing from friends of mine who have had similar things happen that your body just changes over time. That's where I draw the big question mark."

He notices a progressive decline when he's more fatigued, generally, or when he's sleep deprived, feels overtrained, or has had too much caffeine. Taylor has been doing one sport or another since his late teens. At times, he would ski in the winter and transition straight into cycling in the summer. Now he does both, and adds ski mountaineering, alpine touring, and alpine climbing to his list of favorite activities. But he has deliberately backed off the highest intensities of sports.

"For a long time you're operating under the notion that all of this stuff is good for you—you're strong, you're fit, you can do whatever. And when you're in your twenties, you feel fine. But now, you feel little skipped beats or whatever, and maybe the heart just behaves differently. So I don't know what is normal," Taylor says.

Our conversation is filled with questions, a discussion of what is and is not normal. Taylor is asking all the questions, repeatedly stating he's on the pathway of learning more before going to a specialist. But he never relents and says, "You know, you're right. I'm going to make an appointment tomorrow."

Taylor is not alone. Countless people resist what others might consider common sense: seeing a doctor when something seems different. What could be the harm? Why wouldn't you want to understand the situation better and have peace of mind?

Ultimately, the question becomes, why are so many people reluctant to see a doctor in general? Sociologists and clinicians have investigated this question in a range of individuals, from those who don't feel the necessity to those who apparently cannot bear the possibility of bad news.

Studies have shown that people stay away for a number of reasons, including being overly optimistic that they will get better no matter what. But the bottom line for many people is fear: fear of bad news, fear of an uncomfortable test, fear of discussing something intimate.

The American Heart Association has compiled a list of reasons why people often resist going to the doctor, even for an annual physical. It's worth applying those examples to heart health, and, more importantly, to ways to counter those reasons and get yourself or a person you care about to see a doctor.

1. "I don't have a doctor."

Step one toward staying healthy is finding a doctor you trust. But you'll never know if you'll trust one unless you try one. Check your insurance company or local listings for doctors in your area. Call their offices and ask questions, or check around online. It's also a good idea to check with friends and family for recommended doctors.

2. "I don't have insurance."

Everybody should have insurance under the Affordable Care Act. You will have some out-of-pocket costs, of course, but those aren't a reason to avoid getting care.

3. "There's probably nothing wrong."

You may be right, but you're not a doctor. That's why you need one, to obtain certainty. Some serious diseases don't have overt symptoms.

4. "I don't have time."

There are about 8,766 hours in a year. Take two of those hours and see a physician if you suspect a problem, however minor.

5. "I don't want to spend the money."

It makes more sense to spend a little and save a lot than to save a little and spend a lot. If you think visiting a doctor is expensive, consider how expensive it could be if you end up needing an ambulance or taking a trip to a hospital.

6. "Doctors don't do anything."

When you see a barber, you get a haircut. When you see the dentist, your teeth get cleaned. But when you see a doctor, it may seem that he or she just takes notes on your medical history and runs tests. It may seem like you don't get anything, but you do. You get news and knowledge that can bring better health, if you act on it.

7. "I don't want to hear what I might be told."

Your doctor is there to help you. You can deny your reality, but you can't deny the consequences. So be smart: Listen to someone who'll tell you truths you need to hear. Be coachable.

8. "I've got probe-a-phobia."

Wires, scans, ECGs: Visits to the doctor can be intimidating. Remember, though, that your chances of understanding and preventing further damage to your heart are much better if the issue is caught early. It's always worth the exam.

9. "I'd rather tough it out."

You're convinced it'll go away. You assure yourself the issue will pass. "I'm just getting older." "It's only minor." "It's so infrequent." When it comes down to it, there are no good reasons not to see the doctor, only excuses. Don't wait.

7 | Addicted to exertion

CHRIS CASE

PRE-DAWN WAKEUPS—when it's snowing outside. Intervals while on vacation—or Thanksgiving morning. Chasing exercise this way may sound absurd when it's spelled out, but many of us have been driven to even greater lengths in the name of "fitness." Being obsessed with exerting yourself can become a real problem. When it starts to alter how you live your life, it can develop into an exercise addiction.

Could a true addiction have anything to do with the excessive amounts of running, riding, or swimming you do? Could this behavioral addiction be to blame for people developing arrhythmias?

It's worth restating that exercise is extremely beneficial to your general health. But some people take that adage to an unhealthy extreme, believing that if 30 minutes a day is good for you, two hours a day is four times better. The arithmetic, however, does not work in such a linear way.

In fact, according to some studies, 10 percent of high-performance runners, and possibly an equal number of body builders, have an exercise addiction (a condition also referred to as exercise dependence, obligatory exercising, exercise abuse, and compulsive exercise, though no formal diagnosis exists within the scientific community). These individuals are compulsive about doing their exercise of choice, and do it not purely for the love of getting out.

"There is a distinction to be made between the terms 'commitment' and 'compulsion,'" says Duncan Simpson, an associate professor in sports, exercise, and performance psychology at Barry University in Miami. "When we're trying to get people to exercise, we don't worry too much about the reasons, but we do want people to be committed, rather than driven by compulsion, or because of an addiction. Certainly, if you're training for a marathon, you have to be committed."

You can distinguish healthy enthusiasts from exercise addicts by how they shape their lives, says Ian Cockerill, a sports psychologist at the University of Birmingham, England. "Healthy exercisers organize their exercise around their lives, whereas dependents organize their lives 'round their exercise," he says.

Of utmost importance in distinguishing between addicted and nonaddicted exercisers is the difference in incentive for fulfilling planned exercise. Nonaddicted individuals will exercise for a tangible reward such as feeling in shape, looking good, being with friends, staying healthy, losing weight, and so on. The personal experience of the anticipated reward reinforces the exercise behavior. This positive reinforcement helps them maintain their exercise routine since they directly benefit from the activity.

"Of course, we're also dealing with people's perception of what it means to be addicted," Simpson says. "With the vernacular meaning of 'addiction,' it's almost something people use in a positive sense. It's like a cool thing to say. But there is a subset of a large population that is truly addicted."

In that addicted—truly addicted—individual, research has demonstrated the exercise is done in order to avoid negative feelings or withdrawal. For example, the daily run may have become a chore that has to be fulfilled, otherwise an unwanted event would occur, such as an inability to cope with stress, weight gain, or mood swings. Each time a person undertakes the behavior to avoid something negative, the motive acts as negative reinforcement. In short, the person feels he or she *has* to do it, whether the desire to do it is present or not.

This modification of mood is key to the symptoms of true exercise addiction, which is by definition a subclass of behavioral addictions generally. There is a self-medication aspect to whatever discipline(s) the person chooses to pursue, one that feeds into a dangerous cycle whereby addicts no longer exercise for enjoyment, but rather to escape those negative feelings.

The symptoms and consequences of exercise addiction have often been characterized by six common components of addiction: salience (how prominent a role it plays in one's life), mood modification, tolerance, severe withdrawal symptoms (similar to chemical addictions, including alcohol), personal conflict (intra- and interpersonal), and relapse.

Mark Griffiths, a British psychologist from Nottingham Trent University who specializes in addictive behavior, helped create one of the most widely used screening tools in the research area of exercise addiction (Table 7.1). Its popularity is a function of its brevity and excellent psycho-metric properties. That is, it is short, reliable, and has been validated by subsequent testing.[1]

The Exercise Addiction Inventory (EAI) comprises six statements, each corresponding to one of the six symptoms in this "components" model of addiction. Each statement is rated on a 5-point scale ranging from 1 (strongly disagree) to 5 (strongly agree). To be considered at risk for exercise addiction, one must score at or above 24 out of 30.

	Strongly disagree	Disagree	Neither agree nor disagree	Agree	Strongly agree
Exercise is the most important thing in my life.	1	2	3	4	5
Conflicts have arisen between me and my family and/or my partner about the amount of exercise I do.	1	2	3	4	5
I use exercise as a way of changing my mood (e.g., to get a buzz, to escape, etc.).	1	2	3	4	5
Over time I have increased the amount of exercise I do in a day.	1	2	3	4	5
If I have to miss an exercise session, I feel moody and irritable.	1	2	3	4	5
If I cut down the amount of exercise I do and then start again, I always end up exercising as often as I did before.	1	2	3	4	5

TABLE 7.1. Exercise Addiction Inventory and Individual Factor Loadings Using Principal Component Analysis

The six symptoms of Griffiths's components model are worth describing in more detail. First, salience is said to be present when the physical activity or exercise becomes the most important activity in the person's life and he or she becomes totally preoccupied with exercise. Furthermore, exercise dominates the athlete's thinking, feelings (causing urges or cravings for the exercise of choice), and behavior (to the detriment of other social behaviors).[2]

For example, even when addicted individuals are not actually engaged in exercise, they'll be thinking about the next time they can get out for that ride or run. They'll daydream about the exercise during other tasks like driving, eating, and working (or while attending meetings, but really, who hasn't had this particular symptom?). As their planned exercise time approaches, the urge becomes greater and greater. If they aren't able to start on time, anxiety or fear may build inside. Truly addicted exercisers are obsessed with exercise and consumed by the thought of it; regardless of the time of day, place, or activity performed, their minds are preoccupied with exercise during the majority of their waking hours.

Mood modification pertains to the experiences someone will report as a result of partaking in a particular activity. While most healthy people would report a "high" or experience feelings of escape while exercising, addicted exercisers seek to change their mood, but not necessarily for positive reasons. Instead, they seek to avoid negative thoughts and feelings that would arise if they missed out on a session. The fear of guilt or simply not feeling well will drive them to exercise.[3]

Of course, the more you partake of an activity in order to elicit a mood-modifying effect, the greater your tolerance becomes. Thus, more is needed to gain the same results. The runner needs to run longer distances to experience the runner's high, the intense euphoric effect of enthusiastic exercise attributed to the release of endorphins. Similarly, addicted exercisers need progressively greater amounts of exercise to derive the effects once experienced with lesser amounts. That is why individuals addicted to exercise gradually increase the frequency, duration, and intensity of their workouts.[4]

One of the most important symptoms in diagnosing true exercise addiction is withdrawal. And it isn't enough to simply feel glum for a bit when you can't get out. We're talking about severe symptoms. This type of withdrawal refers to unpleasant psychological and physical symptoms that occur when exercise is discontinued or significantly reduced. The most commonly reported are guilt, irritability, anxiety, sluggishness, feeling fat, a lack of energy, and bad mood or depression. The symptoms in addicted individuals will often be severe; they feel miserable and depressed when they can't exercise. Contrast this to the mood of a committed (but not addicted) exerciser who can't get out for that run: He or she may simply feel a void or that something is missing, or have legs that feel tight and antsy. Addicted exercisers *have* to exercise in order to overcome withdrawal symptoms, even at the expense of other important life obligations.[5]

For the addicted, several types of conflict can arise in their lives as a result of their obsession. Interpersonal conflict usually results from neglect of a relationship with friends or family because of the exorbitant amount of time and preoccupation devoted to exercise. Conflict in daily activities arises because of the abnormally high priority given to exercise in contrast to important day-to-day activities like cleaning, home finances, a job, or educational pursuits. Intrapsychic conflict (conflict within the addicted person) occurs when that person realizes fulfilling the need to exercise interferes with other obligations in life, but he or she is unable to reduce the amount of exercise and subsequently experiences a subjective loss of control. In a vicious cycle, the conflict will often lead to additional stress, which compels the person to exercise even more in an effort to relieve that stress.[6]

Finally, we have relapse, the tendency for addicted individuals to revert to unhealthy and excessive exercise after a break, which can be voluntary or involuntary. Maybe they were unable to reduce or cease the unhealthy pattern of exercise, or perhaps an injury led to the same. Once relapse has occurred, the activity resumes and the addicted individuals can often end up exercising as much as (or even more than) they did prior to ceasing exercise. Relapse prevention is one of the greatest challenges in addiction medicine.

Of course, there are a host of other reported symptoms in those afflicted with an exercise addiction, many with severe consequences. These include a loss of control over life activities as well as over the exercise itself, the risk of injury (since addicted exercisers cannot abstain from exercise even if they are injured), denial, and social withdrawal (to avoid criticism). It's interesting to note that because there is no social stigma attached to exercising, such addiction is often given the oxymoronic label of "positive addiction."

Several physical and psychological models attempt to explain why and how people get addicted to exercise. However, none of these models can

explain every case because the trigger, which is usually a highly stressful event in one's life, varies from one person to another. Still, it's worth
considering a few of them in order to better understand the underlying
mechanisms of this behavioral addiction.

A significant number of psychological models are based on "learning theory," wherein both positive reinforcers (for example, a feeling of
euphoria following exercise or muscle growth from exercise) and negative reinforcers (for example, the cessation of unpleasant feelings through
exercise or the avoidance of the presumed negative effect of missed exercise) may be involved in the development and maintenance of compulsive and addictive exercise behavior.

Other research emphasizes the role of "cognitive appraisal mechanisms" in developing patterns of excessive exercise. In this model, the
habitual exerciser uses exercise to cope with stress. The addicted individual learns to depend on exercise in times of stress and then becomes
trapped in a vicious cycle of needing more exercise to deal with the consistently increasing life stress, part of which is caused by exercise itself.

Furthermore, the way in which individuals evaluate themselves can
affect the outcome. For example, the physical sensations experienced
through exercise in people dissatisfied with their bodies or body image
can contribute to the formation of a more positive self-image and self-
assessment. It has also been shown that exercise activities (such as
weightlifting) have a positive effect on body image and self-esteem in
both men and women. Perfectionism, obsessive-compulsive behavior,
and heightened anxiety have also been suggested as determining factors
in exercise addiction.

There are further theories as to the biological and physiological processes involved in the development and maintenance of exercise addiction. As noted earlier, the sensation of the runners' high is often ascribed to the release of beta-endorphins during activity. However, the changes researchers have observed in the levels of this morphine-like compound have been seen in the plasma—a peripheral change. Due to their chemical structure, however, beta-endorphins cannot cross the blood-brain barrier, meaning that changes in levels in the bloodstream may not be accompanied by simultaneous changes in the brain. Despite this issue with the data, some researchers believe that peripheral beta-endorphins (endogenous opiates) are able to work in the brain and produce dependence.

Another physiological explanation is based on the research of Thompson and Blanton from the late 1980s. The researchers argue that regular exercise, especially aerobic exercise, if performed for a sustained period, will result in a lower basal heart rate due to the training adaptation. The adaptation is also accompanied by lower sympathetic activity at rest and lower levels of arousal. Individuals may experience what they perceive as lethargy. According to Thomson and Blanton, this lower level of arousal causes athletes to exercise more in order to increase arousal and feel that they are performing optimally. However, the effects of exercise are temporary. Thus, they may conclude they need to exercise even more to achieve the desired stimulation. Of course, because of training adaptations, they may increase not only the frequency but also the intensity of the exercise.

The "thermogenic regulation hypothesis" is based on the physiological fact that intense physical activity increases body temperature. Warmth in the body may trigger a relaxed state, which, in turn, can reduce anxiety.

Therefore, exercise reduces anxiety and aids in relaxation as a consequence of increased body temperature. Of course, those perks motivate people to exercise often. In this way, people become conditioned to exercise whenever they experience anxiety due to the pleasant psychological and anxiety-relieving effects of exercise. The higher their level of anxiety, the greater their need may become to get out and do their thing. Thus, in stressful situations, the frequency, duration, and intensity of their exercise of choice may progressively increase (as they develop tolerance) to obtain a stronger elixir to stress and anxiety.

As in the beta-endorphin hypothesis of the development of exercise addiction, research has also shown that levels of catecholamines, like beta-endorphins, increase following exercise. This led to the formulation of the "catecholamine hypothesis" in 1977. Catecholamines, among other functions, are involved in both the stress response and the sympathetic response caused by intense exercise. According to the hypothesis, brain catecholaminergic activity is altered through exercise. Since catecholamines are involved in regulating both mood and affect, and also play an important role in the reward system, the changes in brain catecholamine levels following exercise are an appealing explanation for the addictive nature of exercise. However, there is no conclusive evidence to support the hypothesis. As with beta-endorphins, it's unclear whether peripheral changes in catecholamine levels have an effect on brain catecholamine levels or vice versa. Furthermore, it is unclear how catecholamine levels in the brain change during exercise because direct measurement is not possible. Thus, the search for a biological explanation of exercise addiction continues.

With a group of Hungarian colleagues, Griffiths coauthored a nationally representative study examining exercise addiction, using the EAI to survey over 2,700 Hungarian adults aged 18–64 years.[7] Results showed the condition is rare, with 0.5 percent of that population being at risk. In specific groups such as university students, however, figures can be much higher, up to 13 percent. Interestingly, another study that looked at 95 ultramarathoners reported only 3.2 percent (or three individuals) were at risk for exercise addiction.

A 2014 study of 1,285 male and female triathletes using the EAI indicated that 20 percent of triathletes were at risk for exercise addiction (females were slightly more vulnerable).[8] That is actually lower than the percentages found in previous studies. A 2002 study reported 43.3 percent of amateur triathletes were at high risk for addiction, and a 2008 study found that 32.5 percent of the Ironman athletes in their study were at high risk. The 2014 findings also suggested that competing in longer distance races (Olympic, Half-Ironman, and Ironman, specifically) puts triathletes at greater risk for exercise addiction than training for shorter races.

"There was almost like a ceiling effect," says Simpson, a coauthor of the study. "We found this in ultra-runners too. We speculated that the training for the Half-Ironman is not that significantly different from a full triathlon. There's only so much training someone can do in a week."

The researchers found no significant association between the risk of addiction and the number of years someone had participated in the sport. However, as the number of weekly training hours increased, so did a triathlete's risk of exercise addiction.

Though no research has correlated exercise addiction to increases in heart arrhythmias, the fact that many people who suffer from this behavioral addiction tend to continuously ramp up the frequency and intensity of exercise makes it interesting to consider the ramifications. And as mentioned in Chapter 4, research has shown that low self-esteem may lead to higher levels of inflammation, fibrosis, and their end result: arrhythmia.

CASE STUDY
Dave Scott: Atrial flutter, atrial fibrillation
Diagnosed at age 62

CHRIS CASE

IRON MAN. That's the title that has been applied to Dave Scott for decades. A six-time winner of the Ironman World Championship in Kona, Hawaii, Scott defined what it meant to be a triathlete, indeed an athlete, in the 1980s and 1990s. His battles with Mark Allen are the stuff of legend. He was the first person ever inducted into the Ironman Hall of Fame.

In his prime, at the height of the "volume wars" when more was always considered better, his weekly workout totals were staggering: swimming between 25,000 and 30,000 meters, cycling 500 miles, and running between 80 and 90 miles, while also lifting weights three days a week. It amounted to between 40 and 48 hours of exercise in any given week.

Now 62, he's still churning away trying to remain that legendary athlete, though life hasn't been without its scares. In September 2014, after a routine ride with friends on a warm summer day, followed by yard work, Scott sat down to dinner with his partner, Christine.

"I just said, 'Oh my God. Feel this.' It was really racing," Scott says of his heart. "We were kind of concerned. I said, 'God, that thing is really roaring.' We checked, and it was 150 or so. I said, 'That's kind of scary.'"

The next morning he could still feel his heart thumping away in his chest. Nevertheless, he went for his usual Sunday morning run. He ended up stopping repeatedly and walking the last mile home. His morning ended in the urgent care center.

From there, doctors recommended he proceed to the emergency room immediately. He did, and it was quickly determined he was in atrial flutter (the condition where the atria contract rapidly at a regular rate, as opposed to the irregular rhythm of fibrillation, where the atria quiver but do not contract). Measures would need to be taken to reset Scott's heart. He was sedated and cardioverted.

"I came up a little bit later: 'Ta-da! Okay. You're good!'" he says of his return to sinus rhythm.

Since then, Scott has had to face a multitude of challenges, not least of which has been the psychological challenge of facing one's mortality. For someone whom people have elevated as an immortal fitness god, slowing down is a challenge in itself.

I sat down with Scott to discuss life after his initial diagnosis.

You're someone whom people look up to as the epitome of fitness. Is it hard for you to accept what has happened to you? Do you talk about it with people or try to hide the fact?
My first reaction: It kind of pissed me off. "Why me? Really? Me?" Not something that would happen to me. If I ever tell anyone, "I'm not in really good shape," they don't want to hear that. They don't want to believe that. They don't want to recognize that. I'm infallible. "You're Dave Scott. You're always in shape." That particular standard, that aura, has followed me for a long time in my profession. I don't really say anything because I don't want to have to tell people, "Gee, I haven't been doing much because I'm traveling and busy with other stuff. I haven't been working out like I normally do." They don't want to hear that, so it's not a subject I approach.

When it happened to me, I kept thinking, "Wow. How did that happen?" Well, it's kind of the perfect storm that happened. I set myself up for that day. I was aware that a lot of endurance athletes are predisposed to arrhythmias. This long-term, multi-decade overload that we're having. A lot of folks that have done the research and a lot of the medical scientists have told me, "Well, yeah, you dumb shit." The probability of it went up quite a bit based on all that I've done.

I talk about it a lot, about the volume of training people do. I've seen it for a long time, for years. I had a good opportunity in coaching some of the best—Chrissie Wellington and Craig Alexander. There's probably not a single individual between both genders that has come to the sport that doesn't think more is better. "If I can do more, I'm going to be stronger." That was my premise for my initial training. I just want everyone to read about Dave Scott, that he's doing these crazy workouts and this huge volume.

I've been on this warpath well before I had this incident, and I think it's important that I keep talking about it. It's not that I want to avoid it or push it under the carpet. It happened to me, and I'm cognizant that I'm vulnerable and that I feel these heightened periods again. Which makes me mad. I think, "I had one bout. Okay, now I'm done. It's going to go away."

I remember one physician said to me, "Well, you're probably going to die of a blood clot someday. There's a high likelihood of getting a clot, and you'll probably die." [A danger shared by atrial flutter and atrial fibrillation lies in developing clots in the heart that can travel to the brain and cause a stroke. This is because the blood in the atria is not being pumped rapidly, and the surface of this jiggling blood pool can subsequently coagulate.]

Do you think you are addicted to exercise?
Yeah. I think I'm not unusual. I think every endurance athlete likes when you get that endorphin release. It affects your satiety center and makes you feel good, relaxes you. I know when

I've had periods where I have said, "It's all or nothing. . . ." I've had periods like this when I raced and was able to win Ironman. People were going, "Dude, you're just a machine." Many, many times I was depressed. The standard was set so high by myself. If I had [planned] an 11-mile run and I could only do seven, I wouldn't do it.

It's like a reverse drug addict, in some way. You're fueling the psychological part where it truly destroys you, so if I couldn't do it entirely, I wouldn't do it. Then I'd have another day where I wouldn't do it. All of a sudden you kind of beat yourself up thinking, "Oh, gee. I'm worthless now. I can't even get out the door, get my shoes on, to do this." The bar was so high. I had a lot of periods like this in my early career. I finally got to the point [of saying], "Shit, I'll kill myself if I keep doing this." A little bit goes a long ways.

Of course, I talk about this all the time, the psychological part, and getting that endorphin release, and what it takes. Most people will feel better even if they do 20 minutes. Get outside and do 20 minutes, and just move—95 percent of the time, you come back and you're going to feel better. I follow that all the time. It's a mandate for me even when I travel. A lot of times, just being fatigued from the wear and tear of travel, I'll get to some place and I always exercise. Your system's out of whack. I always try to do a little bit. Then, I have days where I don't. But if I have two or three days where I don't . . . whew.

Do you think that your heart condition is directly related to pushing yourself all these years?

Absolutely. No doubt about it. Even in high school, I was the guy who would always do extra. I was the guy who would come in early; I'd always do more repeats. In college I would get frustrated looking at my contemporaries that were loafing on some of the sets and smashing on a couple of the other ones, and they'd blow me away. I'm over there just grinding it out.

I remember in college, it would set me in a psychological tizzy too. Every Tuesday the coach would sit in a chair next to my lane and I'd do a timed 3,000-meter swim. That's like a bad blood draw. You're just sitting there and thinking, "Okay. Can I lock in for 30-plus minutes?" That doesn't sound bad on a bike because you have scenery and so on. With running it's a little bit harder. Swimming, you're just looking at that line. You're not involved with anyone else. You're just trying to hold your 100-meter pace. You're going to do 30 of those 100s as hard as you can, ready to go. I did that.

When I started to do triathlons, I started doing a lot of ocean swims, and I realized I wasn't training as much, swimming-wise. I was stronger, and I was recovering better. I was swimming better post-college. I was beating guys that went to nationals that had annihilated me. There were a lot more variables, but I was holding my own or better than folks that were able to beat me. Then

I realized, after I got to the point of doing all three sports, that when I did have a little bit of recovery, I was a little more resilient.

I was battling Mark [Allen] in 1989, and he beat me that year. Then I had a few injuries, and my two boys were born in 1989 and 1990. Then, I decided to come back when I was 40. I didn't want the schedule that was so big and so massive. I'd go out and ride. Three or four days a week I was on my game. I said, "Man, I feel great." I time-trialed big blocks of time, but it wasn't day-in, day-out. So I found at 40 I was getting stronger. Probably because I was a little wiser. Maybe I didn't realize it because I kept it up.

I'm 62 now. I still trained hard in my 50s. I kept thinking I'd go back to Ironman and do it one more time. I still mentally have the same . . . whatever it is. Stupidity. People say that, or my sister would. Just smashing myself.

But I'm more selective when I kind of recognize it. I ran five and a half miles this morning, lifted weights, and swam about 4,000 meters. There's a group I swim with. I coach a swim class. It's quite popular, and there are a lot of good swimmers. I get in afterward. There's another group. I can kind of tell. I swam very hard yesterday, so I said, "Do I have to kill myself two days in a row?" Part of me is . . . these two other people were beating me. I'm thinking, "Shit. God, they're beating me." Annie, she's a pretty good woman swimmer, and this other guy Craig. I said, "I'm on my game. I should be able to whoop them, and I can."

Part of it was just saying, "What's the point? I'm tired. I didn't sleep well."

Are you nervous about your condition? Or are you just putting it in the back of your mind, denying it? How are you dealing with it?

A little bit of both. Yeah, I'm a little bit nervous about it because some days I feel this sort of heavy feeling, and it takes me longer to warm up. I'm aware that my heart rate seems elevated. It feels as though the depth of the inhale is greater. I feel like I'm at 14,000 feet sometimes. I'm taking these slow inspirations. I feel the pull all the time. I have to warm up at a slower rate, and it seems my body's more receptive to doing that.

But even when I'm swimming, I like to play the game. I'm in there with these elite, competitive people. Part of the game is I want to wear them out. They're 23. I want to beat them.

This kid in my group today, he's 20, and he gave up. I said, "I beat him." Then, I said, "Shit. Now I'll probably have a heart attack." Look what I beat. Smart.

It's a little bit denial because sometimes when I'm in the middle of those workouts, I'm thinking, "Damn, am I destined to have my next episode here right now? Or when I stop and hang on the wall? Or when I finish that hard climb?"

8 | Treatment options for athlete arrhythmia

JOHN MANDROLA

REMEMBER THE FUNDAMENTAL RULE of medicine: Doctors should treat the underlying cause of a person's symptoms. If a patient has a fever caused by a bacterial infection, doctors will use antibiotics to kill the bacteria causing the fever. In the case of chest pain due to a heart attack, doctors will remove blockage from the artery, since that would be the cause of the pain. This concept may sound simple, but it is an important theme to keep in mind as you read the specific options available to treat symptoms of arrhythmia.

Before treatment begins, your doctor needs to take two fundamental steps: first, make a diagnosis, and second, evaluate any associated issues. Let's look at these two before moving on to treatments.

Diagnosis

The first step in the treatment of any heart rhythm problem is getting the correct diagnosis. Doctors approach the treatment of benign premature beats from the atria (PACs) and ventricles (PVCs) differently than they would more serious arrhythmias such as ventricular tachycardia due to heart failure.

When a person complains of an abnormal sensation in the chest, doctors try to record the rhythm during the complaint. It's important to note that the degree of symptoms does not predict the severity of disease. Some patients will complain bitterly over only 100 PVCs daily, while others have no sense that they are having 30,000 PVCs daily. Doctors don't yet understand why people perceive their heart sensations so differently.

What company does the arrhythmia keep?

The second key step to treating heart rhythm disorders is asking what company the arrhythmia keeps. Heart doctors are taught early on in their training to ask, "Does the patient with symptoms of arrhythmia have 'structural' heart disease?"

Sorting out the structural disease question can be as important as getting the right diagnosis. Here's why: An athlete who complains of occasional skipping and jumping of the heartbeat can largely be reassured if the initial tests reveal normal findings. It's common for doctors to tell patients with infrequent symptoms that there is no known cause of their symptoms, but that their heart's electrical and structural condition is good. That's great, because having "no structural heart disease" predicts an excellent outlook.

As we've already seen, doctors determine the structural condition of the heart in various ways. The search begins with the medical history; then the exam and an ECG; and sometimes tests that may include echocardiograms, stress tests, CT scans, nuclear imaging, and MRI scans.

Treating premature heartbeats (PACs and PVCs)

It's not unusual for athletes to experience premature beats. When these beats occur in an otherwise healthy heart, the first and most important treatment is reassurance. Reassurance through information is crucial because premature beats can cause a lot of anxiety, and the anxiety makes the premature beats worse. Before a doctor does an assessment, the patient isn't sure what's going on.

Doctors don't understand why groups of heart cells start to fire prematurely. But one thing is clear: The brain and heart are connected. Something is telling the heart to do this. Being anxious about the skipped beats stimulates the adrenergic nervous system (the fight-or-flight nervous system), which can make premature beats more frequent and more bothersome.

The simple act of reassurance alleviates worry, and less worry means a calmer mind. A calmer mind can lead to a calmer heart rhythm. Patients often tell me their skipped beats got better after they were reassured nothing was wrong. Doctors don't always have to cure with surgery.

A slow resting heart rate creates a favorable milieu for premature beats. The more time that passes between heartbeats, the more opportunity there is for groups of heart cells to fire randomly. At a heart rate of

60 beats per minute, the time between these waves of heart contractions is one second. If the heart rate is 30 beats per minute, it's two seconds.

Doctors will also inquire about precipitating causes in a patient with premature beats. Usually, there's too much of something: too much alcohol, too much emotional or mental stress, too much training, or all of them. Sometimes the contributing factor for premature beats is too little of something: not enough sleep or insufficient recovery between workouts.

Do you notice the theme? Imbalance tends to create an environment for premature beats.

Now, remember the basic principle of medicine: If the cause of the premature beats is too little rest, the treatment is rest. If the cause of the premature beats is a hectic work and training schedule, the best treatment is to make better choices in balancing life's demands. It's unusual for premature beats to occur without a reason, and finding that reason can go a long way toward resolving the issue. If an athlete who is experiencing PACs/PVCs continues to train, there is a possibility the symptoms will worsen. It depends on the underlying cause of the premature beats.

The other thing about premature beats is they tend to go away as mysteriously as they came. The 18th-century French wit and philosopher Voltaire once remarked that the job of a doctor is to humor the patient for as long as it takes nature to fix the problem. Although the culture of modern medicine promotes a quick fix, Voltaire's principle fits nicely with the treatment of premature benign heartbeats.

The main reason for using the stalling techniques of Voltaire is the absence of better options. Take drugs, for instance. The problem with heart rhythm drugs like beta-blockers (inhibitors of the adrenaline receptors), calcium channel blockers (inhibitors of calcium channels), and other sodium and potassium channel blockers are both their lack of efficacy and side effects. (Although one of the side effects, sluggishness, can be unintentionally useful. I've had patients with premature beats tell me they'd rather have occasional skips than be tired all the time from the drugs.)

Doctors may not know the underlying cause of premature beats, but most agree it is rarely a problem with heart cells themselves. Drugs that alter normal function of the ion channels in the heart muscle cells may or may not suppress the beats. And even if drugs do relieve the burden of skips, it's likely the drugs will alter top performance of the heart. All the commonly prescribed heart-rhythm drugs blunt cardiac performance.

Patients and doctors mistakenly call these side effects, but there's nothing side about them. They are effects. When you give a patient a blocker of adrenaline (a beta-blocker), you expect a reduction in maximum heart rate. That reduces performance. When you give a person a calcium channel blocker, you reduce the strength of the heart's contraction. That, too, reduces sports performance. Nonathletic patients may not notice the reduction in cardiac performance from these drugs. But athletes often do.

Two rare conditions of premature beats deserve mention. In the first, the premature beats are numerous (more than 20,000 per day), unrelenting, unresponsive to lifestyle changes or medications, and seem to be originating in a single area. Doctors say these abnormal beats are monomorphic, meaning they have a single morphology or shape.

In these cases, an electrophysiologist may be able to perform a procedure in which a catheter is inserted into the chamber of origin and is then
used to burn (or ablate) the offending cells. This invasive procedure is
called "electrophysiology study and catheter ablation." We will talk more
about ablation in the sections below on atrial fibrillation and atrial flutter.

The other rare situation occurs when PVCs associate with structural
heart disease. In this case, the PVCs are usually a marker for a structural
heart problem such as hypertrophic cardiomyopathy (excess thickening
of the heart), dilated cardiomyopathy (weakened heart muscle), or coronary artery disease. Here, the treatment of the underlying heart condition is critical. In this case, we can view the PVCs as a lifesaver since they
prompted medical evaluation and discovery of a life-threatening problem.

These two situations—unrelenting monomorphic beats or PVCs that
arise from a structural problem—are extremely rare. The vast majority of
premature beats can be managed with time and adjustment of precipitating factors. For athletes, this usually means simply paying more attention
to recovery, sleep, and nutrition.

Treating the patient with atrial fibrillation

The observational evidence we discussed in the previous chapters
strongly suggests that endurance exercise increases the odds of getting
AF. But endurance exercise should not be assumed to be the cause of AF
without a thorough search for common predisposing conditions.

In addition to a history, physical exam, and ECG, a doctor evaluating
a patient with AF will likely do basic laboratory tests (to look for thyroid
problems), and an echocardiogram to sort out the structural condition

of the heart muscle, valves, and chamber sizes. More recently, research has found sleep apnea to be a common precipitating cause of AF. It's true that most athletes don't have the thick body and neck of the typical sleep apnea patient, but it's not uncommon for older and leaner athletes to have an unusual form of sleep apnea. It's worth checking.

Alcohol use is a common predisposing condition. As we've discussed previously, the relationship between alcohol and AF is linear—the more one drinks, the more likely AF is to occur.

Finally, athletes, especially older ones, can develop high blood pressure, which is a clear precipitator of AF.

If a predisposing condition is found, treatment of that problem can lead to elimination of AF. Before we describe specific treatments, though, let's reiterate the value of getting an accurate diagnosis.

AF is defined as more than 30 seconds of an irregularly irregular (chaotic) rhythm. The first question to ask your doctor is whether he or she is sure the problem is AF. Other supraventricular (north of the ventricle) rhythm problems can mimic AF. Atrial flutter and atrial tachycardia can be misdiagnosed as AF. This is not an academic distinction—the treatments for these problems differ greatly from the treatment for AF.

Another common pitfall of diagnosis comes when short "runs" of arrhythmia are overdiagnosed as AF. Sometimes a long-term ECG monitoring is read as saying the patient had "seven seconds of AF." This is a misdiagnosis, or overdiagnosis, because the correct diagnosis of AF requires 30 seconds of an irregular chaotic rhythm.

Now, let's assume the diagnosis is accurate and there are no underlying structural causes for the AF. What are the specific treatments?

Detraining

Detraining—backing off from regular, intense exercise—is the first intervention to consider in treating AF in an athlete. That may sound terrible
to an exercise fanatic, of course, but it is a safe and easy experiment that
can lead to a resolution of symptoms.

In Chapter 4, we described the evidence whereby training effects
could induce AF. If training stress is the cause of AF, the rules of good
medical practice say that the treatment should target the cause. Do you
remember the experiments on mice from Montreal? In that experiment,
detraining reversed the mice's susceptibility to provoked AF.

Sadly, we cannot cite any definitive medical studies that show detraining reverses AF in humans. They don't exist. We do know, however, that
detraining will likely result in slightly higher resting heart rates. That may
be important for AF because with less time between beats, there will be
fewer chances for PACs to initiate the AF.

Detraining may also result in reversal of the normal hypertrophy of
the heart. That, too, may help promote a more stable rhythm.

Most importantly, though, a trial of detraining is safe. Not training for
a while won't kill you, and an overarching rule of good medical practice is
to first, do no harm.

Detraining does not mean that you have to go from training 15 hours
a week to zero. But you do need to back off considerably. What does that
mean, precisely? Well, the literature is sparse; we can't quote any proven
protocols of detraining. All we have to go on is logic. And logically, if you
are putting in 15 hours, you should cut that at least in half as a trial. If you
don't see a difference, try cutting by half again.

Before you throw this book down in disgust, consider what a shot at detraining means relative to the other options. Once you read the next section on drugs and procedures, mapping out your own reduced exercise routine, in consultation with your doctor, may look better than it does now.

Stress reduction

There is less science to cite connecting stress and atrial fibrillation. But any kind of stress can lead to increased arrhythmias: Marital problems, difficulty with children, grief from the loss of a parent, stress at work, and declining personal health are just a few examples.

Researchers from the University of Kansas studied an unconventional treatment approach to AF—yoga.[1] They enrolled 52 patients with symptomatic AF into a clinical trial in which patients in the active arm received twice-weekly yoga sessions. Over the course of three months, patients in the yoga group, when compared with the standard care group, reported fewer symptomatic and nonsymptomatic AF episodes, lower scores on anxiety measures, and higher scores on vitality and general health. Blood pressure, too, fell in the yoga group.

Swedish researchers found similar findings in a study of 80 patients with symptomatic AF.[2] They noted drops in heart rate and blood pressure, and improvements in quality of life. Notably, the drop in blood pressure observed in both these yoga trials (6–8 mmHg) is similar to that seen in many of the drug studies.

Two small studies aren't enough to prove yoga eliminates AF. But think of these trials from a mechanistic vantage point. If yoga can relieve symptoms of AF and reduce objective measures of stress (heart rate and blood pressure), that, at least, suggests stress and anxiety may have a significant role in AF.

Stroke prevention

When AF occurs, the number one complication to worry about is stroke. In large studies of populations, the presence of AF associates with a higher probability of stroke.

Most experts believe the increase in stroke risk stems from stasis of blood in the fibrillating atria. When an atrium fibrillates, it does not properly contract. Blood doesn't flow through the atria as vigorously as it should, which causes clots to form. These clots can travel into the ventricles and then out into the body and brain.

But stasis is not the only factor behind the increased risk of stroke in patients with AF. Fibrillating atria lead to release of chemical factors that actually make the blood stickier, which further promotes clot formation. The "coagulation cascade" is a complicated symphony in our bodies, constantly balancing the level of clotting factors in the blood that help protect the body from bleeding. Too much clotting can lead to unwanted clots; too little clotting can lead to bleeding.

Studies of drugs that block the normal clotting system add to the evidence that clots are an important cause of stroke in patients with AF. Lots of people call these drugs blood thinners, but that's not accurate; the drugs do not affect the viscosity of the blood. Instead, these drugs inhibit different clotting factors in the blood, tilting the coagulation cascade slightly away from clotting.

The most common and well known of these clot-blocking drugs is warfarin (Coumadin). (From 2006 to 2016, the Food and Drug Administration approved four new drugs that also inhibit the normal clotting system. These drugs include dabigatran/Pradaxa, rivaroxaban/Xarelto, apixaban/Eliquis, and edoxaban/Savasya. This class of drugs is called "new oral anticoagulants," or NOACs.)

The warfarin/Coumadin studies, which were mostly conducted in the 1990s, showed that when risk factors such as older age, high blood pressure, diabetes, heart failure, blood vessel disease, or a previous history of stroke showed up in people with AF who took clot-blocking drugs, those patients had a lower likelihood of stroke compared with patients who took a placebo or aspirin. AF patients with no risk factors, however, have a yearly risk of stroke of well under 1 percent. That's not much more than people of the same age without AF. As the number of risk factors increases (old age plus high blood pressure, for example), so does the risk of stroke. When people accumulate more than two risk factors, nearly all doctors agree that the net benefit of clot-blocking drugs outweighs the increased risk of bleeding. It's not a black-and-white decision, though.

Doctors estimate the untreated stroke risk (for patients not on anti-coagulant drugs) with an algorithm called the CHADS-VASC score. It's based on points. One point is given for Congestive heart failure (or simply a weak heart), one point for High blood pressure, one point for Age greater than 65, one point for Diabetes, two points for previous Stroke, one point for Vascular disease (like coronary disease or carotid disease), two points for Age greater than 75, and one point in the sex category (SC) for female gender.

Northern European countries keep national health registries. Using information from these huge databases in which one can search for the health characteristics of patients (that is, whether they have AF, are taking an anticoagulant drug, or have had a stroke), doctors can estimate the stroke risk of different levels of CHADS-VASC score. The higher the score, the higher the risk of stroke and the more likely the benefit of clot-blocking drugs.

The use of drugs that block clotting has the downside of increasing the chance of bleeding. It's an easy decision not to use these drugs in low-risk patients with AF; the risk of bleeding outweighs the benefits. Likewise, it's an easy decision to use these drugs in patients with a very high risk of stroke; stroke prevention outweighs the risk of bleeding. The gray area exists in the intermediate-risk patients—those with one or two risk factors.

The good news for athletes is that training helps prevent high blood pressure, diabetes, and blood vessel disease. Athletes, especially those under the age of 65, often do not have enough of these risk factors to warrant the use of clot-blocking drugs.

A quick word on aspirin. We can make it simple. There is no compelling evidence that aspirin reduces the risk of stroke in patients with AF. In fact, European guidelines recommend against aspirin use for stroke prevention for AF. American guidelines give aspirin a lukewarm recommendation, saying it may reduce the risk of stroke—but much less so than clot-blocking drugs.

AF drugs

Doctors use two types of drugs for the treatment of AF. The distinction turns more on the purpose of the drugs rather than their chemical makeup.

The first type, rate-controlling drugs (also referred to as AV-node blockers, AV-node antagonists, or AV-node modulators), act on the AV node. These chemicals have little effect on the atrial muscle cells, so they don't necessarily prevent AF. The drugs slow the pulse rate in AF by slowing conduction in the heart from north (atria) to south (ventricle) through the AV node.

The two most common rate-controlling drugs are beta-blockers and calcium channel blockers. Beta-blockers tend to end in –*lol*. Examples include metoprolol, atenolol, and carvedilol. There are only two useful calcium channel blockers, diltiazem and verapamil. Digoxin is an old rate-controlling drug that is rarely used for AF in patients without heart failure.

In nonathletic patients, rate-control drugs are used to slow the rate of AF because sustained heart racing—lasting days to weeks—can weaken the heart muscle. Doctors call this problem "tachycardia-mediated cardiomyopathy." Basically, it's the equivalent of constantly driving your family sedan around at 5,000 rpm; it will be fine for a while but will eventually break down.

Athletes with AF rarely suffer from the problem of persistently high heart rates. Fitness gained from training induces higher vagal tone, which acts to slow conduction through the AV node during AF. What's more, most athletes have the intermittent form of AF, and so sustained heart racing occurs rarely.

One of the big problems for athletes with AF, however, is a high heart rate during exercise. The challenge in using rate-controlling drugs to suppress exercise-induced heart racing is that the drugs exert their effect all day. When an athlete is not exercising, rate-control drugs will slow the athlete's already slow resting heart rate even further (predisposing him or her to fatigue and dizziness due to excessively slow heart rates). And, of course, the drugs reduce performance by lowering heart rate when the athlete is exercising, too.

The second type of AF drugs are called rhythm-control drugs. These agents act on the ion channels that control activation and relaxation of the heart muscle cells themselves. They break down into categories based on the channels they block.

The sodium channel blockers include propafenone and flecainide; the potassium channel blockers include sotalol and dofetilide (not available in Europe). Dronedarone and amiodarone, which comprise a third group of rhythm-control drugs, act on multiple ion channels.

Medical trials that evaluated the effectiveness of these drugs never enrolled athletes alone. They can still be used in athletes, but there is no definitive evidence that they solve athletes' particular problems with AF. Moreover, the use of these rhythm-control drugs comes with many warnings. The great paradox of rhythm-control drugs is that they can, in some cases, make the rhythm worse, a condition that doctors call "pro-arrhythmia." That refers to a situation in which the effect of the ion-channel blockade can help another arrhythmia develop—sometimes a more ominous rhythm.

Pro-arrhythmia

The least dangerous effect of rhythm-control drugs is their slowing of the heart rate. That can induce fatigue or dizziness but rarely leads to serious complications.

A more hazardous pro-arrhythmia effect, particularly from the sodium channel blockers, is the organization of atrial fibrillation into atrial flutter. Although this sounds like a good thing, since atrial flutter is more organized than the chaos of AF, it's not. The problem with a sodium-channel-blocker-induced atrial flutter becomes apparent when the athlete exercises. It's beyond the scope of this book to explain the why and how, but the net effect is that the athlete taking a sodium channel blocker who develops atrial flutter while exercising can develop rates of greater than 250 beats per minute. That can lead to collapse. Rich Peverley, a professional hockey player who collapsed on the ice and was shocked out of an arrhythmia during a game, is widely believed to have suffered from extremely high heart rates during an AF-drug-induced atrial flutter.

Pro-arrhythmia from sodium channel blockade is unfortunate, because these drugs do a nice job of suppressing AF in nonathletes with intermittent AF. They do a decent job of suppressing premature beats, too.

One way around the issue of rapid conduction of atrial flutter is to add a rate-controlling drug. Nonathletic patients do reasonably well with this two-drug approach. Athletes, however, rarely tolerate two drugs that slow heart rate and inhibit performance.

Another workaround for the use of sodium channel blockers in athletes is to use them only when needed. Doctors call this the "pill-in-the-pocket" approach. It's modeled after a 2004 study in the *New England Journal of Medicine* in which high doses of these drugs were used to terminate recent-onset AF in outpatients.[3]

The advantage of using drugs only during the AF episode is that it minimizes exposure to the drug. The problem, of course, is that if you don't take the drug on a daily basis, it provides no AF prevention. The other problem with the pill-in-the-pocket approach is that an athlete who takes a high dose of the drugs and then goes training could be at risk for rapid conduction of atrial flutter.

The most dangerous pro-arrhythmia effect comes into play with drugs that block potassium channels. Here's the problem: Rhythm drugs exert their effects in the atria—and in the ventricles.

Potassium channel blockers slow the time it takes the heart to relax; on the ECG, this interval is called the "QT interval (Figure 8.1). It's

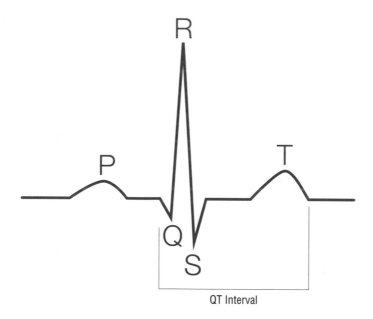

FIGURE 8.1. The QT interval on a normal ECG trace. The entire interval from P to T equals one cardiac cycle; see also Figure 1.6.

pretty easy to measure. Blocking potassium channels is precarious—a little blockade helps prevent arrhythmia, but too much can cause a lethal brand of ventricular tachycardia known by its French name "torsades de pointes," or twisting of the points, due to its distinct appearance on the ECG. It is a malignant arrhythmia because it can lead to sudden death. This severe downside, along with the fact that most potassium blockers profoundly slow the heart rate, makes these drugs of little use to the athlete with AF.

Catheter ablation

The many negative effects of drug therapy have led to the increasing use of procedures to control AF. Most common is catheter ablation.

In this procedure, the doctor uses catheters with electrodes inserted through blood vessels in the groin (or arms or neck, in some cases) and then into the heart. These catheters are used to map the origin of the arrhythmia and then another catheter is used to deliver a three- to four-millimeter-sized burn that kills those few problem cells. The small burn does not damage the heart, but it stops the firing of an abnormal circuit. Burning may sound crude, but in fact ablation is an elegant procedure that offers a total cure when the problem arises from one spot.

In the late 1990s, a group of heart rhythm doctors from Bordeaux, France, first described a special sort of AF that seemed to be occurring from within the pulmonary veins.[4] Until this seminal discovery, most people thought of the pulmonary veins as simple pipes that carried oxygenated blood from the lungs to the heart. The French group showed that these veins could harbor a focus of a rapid irregular rhythm that looked like AF. The discovery that this single focus from within the vein could be ablated with a catheter ignited the practice of AF ablation.

The French researchers combined their electrical observations with previous anatomic observations showing that the pulmonary veins are actually wrapped in heart muscle cells. This led to the concept that the pulmonary veins harbored the cause of, or at least the triggers for, AF.

Two new discoveries soon dampened the initial excitement that AF could be as curable as other focal arrhythmias. The first was that burning within the veins caused an injury reaction that led to severe constriction of the vein, which then caused terrible breathing problems. Doctors call this complication "pulmonary vein stenosis."

The second problem had to do with the fact that humans have four pulmonary veins. Patients who had an ablation around one pulmonary vein would often later develop triggers from within the three other pulmonary veins. Sadly, AF almost always arises from more than one area.

Within a few years following the discoveries in France, the typical AF ablation procedure morphed into one using multiple ablation lesions to build wide circles around the orifices of all the pulmonary veins. The best way to think about pulmonary vein isolation (PVI) with ablation is to envision it as an electric fence made by many point-to-point burns (Figure 8.2). Even though AF can occur from within the vein, the "fence" prevents it from getting out to the heart. These burns don't affect blood flow, only the electrical conduction of signals. As you remember, cell-to-cell conduction requires live cells. The burn kills the cells and thus forms a barrier to electrical conduction.

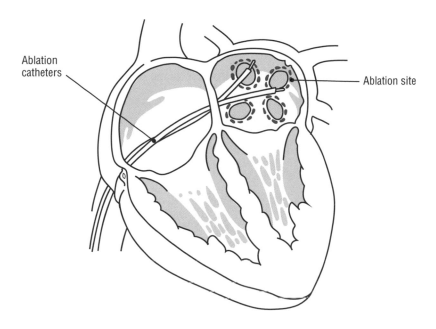

Ablation catheters

Ablation site

FIGURE 8.2. Pulmonary vein ablation

In recent years, cryoballoon techniques have allowed doctors to electrically isolate pulmonary veins with single-shot circular freezes. In this procedure, a double balloon is threaded into place, and the inner balloon then gets a shot of nitrous oxide, which transforms from a liquid to a gas at about –80°F. (An alternative technology uses liquid nitrogen.) The desired outcome is the same as with ablation: The muscle sleeves surrounding the veins no longer connect with the atrium and, thus, if AF originates from within the veins, it cannot propagate into the left and right atria.

A large study with a cool name, the Fire and Ice trial, showed equivalent results with either point-to-point radiofrequency (fire) ablation

or cryoballoon (ice) ablation for the electrical isolation of the pulmonary veins.[5]

If only AF ablation therapy were as easy as electrically disconnect-
ing the pulmonary veins. Despite many improvements in catheter design
and mapping techniques, single-procedure long-term (five-year) success
rates for AF ablation hover around 50 to 60 percent. And as many as one
in three patients require multiple ablation procedures.

Moreover, AF ablation is a big procedure. Most hospitals use general
anesthesia, which despite its common use is no small matter. Doctors
place multiple large-bore intravenous (IV) lines in the leg veins. Major
complications occur at a rate of 2–5 percent, and they are indeed major:
They include stroke, perforation of the heart, life-threatening damage
to the esophagus, paralysis of the diaphragm, stenosis of the pulmonary
veins, and injury to the blood vessels in the leg.

Experts in electrophysiology debate almost every aspect of AF ablation. They contest what defines success; right now, even 30 seconds of
nonsymptomatic AF is considered a procedure failure. That may seem
nitpicky, but if AF is still present even if not felt, the risk of stroke could
be increased. That's why experts have been strict about defining AF.

The stroke question is debated, too. For instance, experts argue about
whether ablating AF reduces the risk of stroke. Right now, there is no
medical evidence that successful ablation accomplishes that. You'd think
it would, but it's not known for sure. Two major studies are currently
looking at this question, but enrollment is slow because patients referred
to expert centers due to AF usually want ablation. What's more, these
studies will require long-term follow-up. Results will take years.

Should an athlete with AF undergo ablation?

A few small studies have reported ablation outcomes in athletes. In 2010 Spanish investigators compared outcomes of ablation in patients with intermittent AF who had a history of endurance exercise against a group who did not.[6] Success rates were similar for athletes and nonathletes after the first AF procedure. When they looked at outcomes after multiple procedures, 81 percent of athletes, versus 63 percent of nonathletes, remained free of AF. The difference reached statistical significance, but this study recruited only 182 patients from 2003 to 2006.

A year later, a Belgian group reported AF ablation outcomes in 94 runners, cyclists, swimmers, and rowers.[7] They used a sample of 41 nonathletes as controls. After an average follow-up of three years, this experienced group of AF experts reported only 48 percent and 46 percent success rates after the first ablation procedure. Final outcomes after multiple procedures increased to 87 percent and 84 percent in the respective groups.

One could interpret these studies in two ways. The first is that athletes do equally well with ablation and the other is that athletes do just as poorly as nonathletes.

Athletes with atrial fibrillation face a tough decision. It's a gamble. To benefit from the procedure, the patient has to accept the risk that the procedure will not work or could cause a complication. And even with successful elimination of AF episodes, it's not clear that performance remains the same. Maybe it does; we just don't know.

If that weren't enough, it's possible that returning to heavy training and competition may incite other areas of the atria—outside the pulmonary veins—to trigger or sustain AF.

All of these "maybes" and "possibilities" are frustrating to those suffering from AF, who want a clear course of action. Unfortunately, that is the nature of what we currently know about AF. It's also why a trial of lifestyle intervention and detraining may look more reasonable, once you consider the complications from drugs and the modest performance results and risks of ablation.

Atrial flutter

Atrial flutter and AF often occur together. (Patients usually can't tell whether they are in flutter or fibrillation.) Cardiologists use the term "flutter" to mean a fast *and* organized rate in the atria. Usually, atrial flutter consists of a circular rhythm around the right atrium.

The atrial rate in flutter is usually 240 to 300 beats per minute. Conduction to the ventricle, through the AV node, varies but is usually a ratio of the atrial rate. For instance, the classic flutter rate is 300 beats per minute in the atrium and 150 beats per minute in the ventricle. The ventricle determines the pulse, so a 2:1 flutter is typically 150 beats per minute. Remember the beautiful AV node; it protects us from the 300-bpm flutter.

Since atrial flutter causes a fast rhythm in which the atria and ventricles are not in sync, patients usually feel some sort of symptoms. Athletes with atrial flutter will often report that their tolerance of exercise is severely reduced.

Drugs rarely work for atrial flutter. It's a bit beyond the scope of this book to explain why, but it has to do with the organized nature of flutter. Plus, the same issues with drug therapy in athletes with AF apply here: namely, endurance athletes don't tolerate these drugs very well.

The good news for athletes is that the typical atrial flutter is much more easily ablated than AF. Luckily, in the right atrium, part of the circular flutter goes through an isthmus between the entry of the inferior vena cava (IVC) and the tricuspid valve. The anatomy is not as important as the idea that this 20-mm isthmus is easily reached with a catheter, and it is a thick area of the heart that is safe to ablate. Once ablated, the electrical circuit can no longer pass around the right atrium, and the atrial flutter is fixed.

One big problem remains: Patients with atrial flutter can also have AF. Some people think the left atrial source of AF and the right atrial source of flutter are two sides of the same coin. Different studies produce different absolute percentages, but approximately one-third to one-half of patients who have had successful flutter ablation go on to develop AF. This is an important observation, because doctors can advise patients who have had successful flutter ablation to avoid things that cause AF— alcohol, excessive training, and so on.

Cardioversion

Cardioversion is a procedure in which a doctor delivers a high-voltage shock from two pads placed on the front and back of a patient's chest. The voltage stops the heart momentarily; the heart then resets to a regular (sinus) rhythm. It's a technique that can be used for the treatment of both AF and atrial flutter.

Of course, cardioversion requires that patients be heavily sedated or put under anesthetic. Nobody can tolerate the shock while awake. The instantaneous success rate of cardioversion approaches 100 percent. The problem with the technique is that it doesn't change the underlying cause of the arrhythmia. Without treating the cause, recurrence of the arrhythmia is likely.

Doctors use cardioversion for multiple reasons. One is to provide relief to the patient. Another is to see how bothersome the arrhythmia becomes. If the patient feels better after cardioversion has restored regular rhythm, that helps prove that the AF or flutter caused his or her complaints. If, on the other hand, a patient has cardioversion, remains in regular rhythm, and then reports still feeling fatigued or tired, it wasn't the abnormal rhythm causing the problem. This happens more than you think. Most nonathletic patients don't feel their AF.

Cardioversions have a good safety record. The most devastating complication of shocking the heart is stroke. Doctors prevent this by using clot-blocking drugs in the weeks or months leading up to and following the procedure.

Treating the patient with ventricular tachycardia

The approach to treating the athletic patient with ventricular tachycardia depends on the company the arrhythmia keeps. Let's start with the worst-case scenario. Athletes who have a racing heartbeat due to VT *and* structural heart disease should stop training, period. They should see an electrophysiologist as soon as possible. VT due to conditions such as hypertrophic cardiomyopathy (excess thickening of the heart muscle), dilated cardiomyopathy (weakened heart muscle), or arrhythmogenic RV cardiomyopathy (ARVC) can be life-threatening. Remember the discussion in Chapter 4 of the causes of sudden death during competition? For athletes under the age of 35, those diseases were the likely causes.

Within the larger setting of structural heart disease, arrhythmia is simply a manifestation of the underlying disease. The treatment of these conditions focuses on keeping the person alive rather than worrying too much about sports performance. All cases are different, but doctors often use a combination of drugs and an implantable cardiac defibrillator (see Chapter 9).

Ventricular tachycardia not due to structural heart disease

Fortunately, "normal-heart" VT is more common in athletes. Determining whether this condition is present relies on an accurate diagnosis (by recording the rhythm) and an assessment for structural disease by means of various testing and scanning methods.

Let's say the problem is a rapid racing of the heart from one source in the ventricle, and the rest of the heart is normal. This is called a monomorphic VT—it emanates from one spot.

The most common area involved in this type of VT is the right ventricle, near the outflow tract under the pulmonic valve, which separates the right ventricle from the pulmonary artery. Doctors call these arrhythmias right ventricular outflow tract ventricular tachycardia (RVOT-VT). They are usually sensitive to adrenaline, and therefore symptoms usually occur with exercise.

No one understands why rogue cells in this area decide to fire up. There are theories, but as many nonathletes get this condition as athletes.

The good news is that if the VT is coming from one area and there is no structural heart disease, a specialist can perform an electrophysiology study, map the area, and then ablate it. The procedure has risks, but it can be curative. In many cases, athletes can, after a few weeks of recovery, return to full-gas competition. Success rates and return to full activity after ablation for normal-heart VT are high, greater than 80 percent.

In nonathletes with normal-heart VT, doctors might offer a trial of drug treatment. Many nonathletic patients with these adrenaline-sensitive arrhythmias can be easily controlled with beta-blockers. But, as we've discussed previously, athletes don't often tolerate beta-blockers.

VT in the "normal heart" can also originate from the left ventricle, usually near the fascicles that are part of the His-Purkinje network. These fascicular VTs, like the RVOT-VT, can also be successfully mapped and ablated.

CASE STUDY
Paul Ernst: Heart failure due to dilated cardiomyopathy
Diagnosed at age 59

CHRIS CASE

WHEN PAUL ERNST first moved to Colorado, he quickly got involved in the outdoors and hiking, and ultimately took up cross-country ski racing. He had a knack for the ski motion and soon learned he was pretty good at it. What you're good at, he says, you do a lot of. From the time he was 30, he started winning masters national championship events, from 15- and 30-kilometer events up to 50-kilometer marathon races.

He continued to compete and improve relative to his peers into his 40s. A VO_2max test (a measure of a person's aerobic fitness) when he was 49 revealed it to be 68 milliliters of oxygen per kilogram of body weight per minute—very high for someone his age. (A figure above 45 is considered excellent for a 40-year-old.)

From about age 50, he started noticing what he now describes as palpitations. Some victims of these occurrences interpret them as skipped beats, but for Ernst they felt like a rocking motion in his chest. It wasn't the first time he had experienced severe bouts of feeling stale for weeks at a time, but this time there was a physical symptom as well.

He now knows that his lack of oomph resulted from over-training. At the time, Ernst's work as an insurance broker gave him wide flexibility in when to train. He'd regularly make his sales pitch to doctors while they skied side by side.

Then came his moment of revelation. Ernst was skiing at Devil's Thumb Ranch in Tabernash, Colorado, on a cold, dreary day. The tracks hadn't been laid very well. He had a few coffees because he just couldn't get himself going. He was churning along when suddenly he experienced what felt like his heart rocking side to side in his chest.

"I thought, 'I'm dying. I just feel like I'm dying. My life is coming out of me.' I just chalked it up to a bad attitude on a gloomy day," he says.

Shortly after that incident, Ernst learned of a study of fitness in seniors at the University of Colorado, and he was interested in the $100 payment as well as the science. "They popped me on the treadmill and said, 'Oh, your VO_2max is pretty good. It's around 52.' I said, 'Fifty-two? It was 68 a year ago!'" Ernst concluded his scores were dropping much faster than might be expected on a normal aging curve. He was alarmed.

Next he underwent an ECG.

"I see these spikes swinging up," he remembers. "'Oh, those are just PVCs. They don't mean anything,' the doc said. Now, I know that they do mean something." He quit racing. He was in an all-or-nothing state of mind: If he couldn't win, he wasn't going to race. But he continued to train pretty hard; he says he was trying to keep his weight down and stay as fit as possible.

But the decline did not slow. From one year to the next, he lost more and more capacity and experienced more frequent palpitations. Around this time, Ernst learned of his friend Mike Endicott's near-death experience at Devil's Thumb (see Chapter 4). He says now he didn't really understand what Endicott was telling him: a fit guy dying in the woods while doing what he loved.

Six months later, Ernst knew exactly what Endicott meant and felt he was on his way to the same fate. "I'm getting out of breath on the stairs. I'm thinking, 'I'm a national champion and I'm struggling on the stairs. What's going on here?'" he says.

After seeing a cardiologist and undergoing an echocardiogram and stress test, he went for a cross-country ski. Of course! When he returned home, a message on his answering machine shocked him into acknowledging the significance of his condition. "Get in here right now. You've had a massive heart attack," he remembers it saying. A return to the doctor revealed he hadn't had a massive heart attack, after all, but he soon learned of his diagnosis: heart failure due to dilated cardiomyopathy.

It is the most common type of cardiomyopathy. It mostly occurs in adults aged 20 to 60, and it affects men more than women. Dilated cardiomyopathy affects both the ventricles and atria, often starting in the left ventricle, the heart's main pumping chamber. The heart muscle begins to dilate (stretch and become thinner), in turn causing the chamber to enlarge. The problem often spreads to the right ventricle and then to the atria as the disease gets worse. Eventually, the heart muscle reaches its capacity, following the so-called Frank-Starling law.

When the chambers dilate, the heart muscle doesn't contract normally, and in turn, the heart can't pump blood very well. Over time, the heart becomes weaker, and heart failure can occur, as in the case of Ernst. Dilated cardiomyopathy can also lead to heart valve problems, arrhythmias, and blood clots in the heart.

"'Here, take some pills, take these beta-blockers and ACE inhibitors, and don't push yourself too hard,' they told me," Ernst says. Eight months later, on October 8, 2007, while out on his roller skis, he collapsed in the street. He woke up a week later in the ICU.

From rereading the medical logs from his ambulance ride and time in the emergency room, Ernst learned it took 11 shocks and 40 minutes to reestablish a normal sinus rhythm in his heart. Another indicator of how poorly his heart was pumping showed that the ejection fraction (EF) of blood from his heart was seriously low. (If you took a flexible 100-milliliter ketchup bottle and gave it a hard squeeze and saw that 40 milliliters remained in the bottle, you can say you ejected 60 percent of the contents.

That's the ejection fraction. And 55 to 60 percent represents a normal, strong, working heart. When Ernst was initially diagnosed, his EF measured in the high 30s, an indication of heart failure. It rose slightly while on drugs but plummeted into the 20s when he was being salvaged in the ICU.)

Ultimately, the cardiomyopathy was the cause of the fibrillation that sent Ernst to the ground. Because of the cardiomyopathy and the constraints of the heart, it overfills. Like a balloon stretched to bursting with blood, it rebounds harder. In turn, that rebound mechanism stores the energy and puts more into the next beat. Eventually it can stretch too far, surpassing the elastic limit, and the heart doesn't get all the rebound energy back. Then it becomes a slack bag that's overfilling and not coming back to its original position the way it should.

Ernst's arrhythmia was precipitated by the overly stretched muscle, and seems to have originated in the right ventricle. He would remain in the hospital for two and a half weeks.

Like others, he didn't back off as much as he should have. He continued to try to be active, even climbing some of Colorado's "fourteeners," mountains that reach at least 14,000 feet. A month after he left the hospital, doctors implanted an ICD in his chest, telling him, "You're on your way; you can make a comeback," he says. "They didn't really give me much direction. I'm thinking, 'I'm an athlete; I know how to rehab.'"

He wore a heart rate monitor to keep things under 120 beats per minute, as he was told to do. Like Endicott, however, it wasn't long before he experienced something shocking. First, it was a spontaneous bout of elevated heart rate that he thought was going to lead to the ICD resetting his heart. It never happened, but while on a walk with his wife he had to lie in a pile of leaves to finally bring his heart rate under control.

"A week later, I'm on the treadmill talking to the woman next to me and I'm probably maybe as high as 120, and all of a sudden it's like a bomb going off," he says. "There's a bright light and a bang and I feel like I've been hit with a baseball bat. I just spat off the treadmill. The thing fired with no warning. Wow, that's really something."

From then on, he went into a period of increasingly frequent shocks. "I would say the first one was interesting and after that, they weren't a whole lot of fun," he says. He went through the better part of a year getting shocked, while doctors recommended he have an ablation. Eventually, he relented. Unfortunately, after putting him to sleep and spending some four hours trying to induce VT, the doctors were unable to elicit the arrhythmia.

Life rolled on. Then one day, while playing soccer with an at-risk second grader at a local school, he got a shock on the playground. The young boy had to run and get help as Ernst lay on the ground and entered an electrical storm.

Ernst knew what this meant, since he had seen Endicott in the hospital after his storm. ("It's like he did two rounds with Mike Tyson," Ernst says of seeing Mike in the hospital.)

"The hell. I thought, 'I don't know if can go through 20 or 30 of these.' I was on the ground praying and mercifully after the sixth shock, it stopped," he remembers. It turned out the device's initial trigger was appropriate, but due to its configuration, it was misreading subsequent signals. The next five shocks were dubbed inappropriate.

"I was turning into a basket case," he says. "I would twitch at night. Sometimes I'd wake up screaming and my wife would say, 'You were in shock,' because she could feel it. I was dreaming. In other words, my brain was getting programmed. I was having phantom shocks. I couldn't tell you a real one from the dreamt one. Then you get scared to go to bed because the ones in the middle of the night are the worst. You're disoriented."

It was time for another ablation, this time while Ernst was awake.

The mapping of his heart was something Ernst described as "interesting." "They're running your heart rate up and down the flagpole trying to induce VT. The electrophysiologist managed to get a three-second burst. He says, 'Nah, it's not really good enough to map but I can guess. Do you want me to ablate it anyway?' I said, 'Yeah, I can't live like this. Do something. I want to walk out of here different,'" he remembers.

That night, ablation completed, he went into VT in the ICU. The next morning, the doctor actually recommended Ernst be put on the transplant list. They also discussed a potent anti-arrhythmic drug, amiodarone. It's exceedingly toxic. But at that point, Ernst was willing to try it. "The doctor said, 'You know that can kill you.' I said, 'I don't care.'" He spent a year on amiodarone without ever experiencing a shock.

(Amiodarone acts by shutting down multiple ion channels in the heart. There are some anti-arrhythmics that act on potassium channels, some on calcium, and others on sodium. Amiodarone shuts down everything. It's a shotgun approach. For it to function effectively, it must achieve systemic saturation. Initially, a patient is titrated with the drug in a hospital. In Ernst's case, that took over three days, while his blood pressure and other vital signs were monitored. Then he took an oral maintenance dose, and would see a pulmonologist, an eye doctor, and other physicians to monitor his physiological functions for side effects that can affect the lungs and eyes.)

A year later, Ernst showed elevated liver enzymes and had to be taken off amiodarone. His worst fear was that he'd go right back to being shocked. But it never happened. He's now five years shock-free. The ablation may have worked after all.

But his heart was damaged enough after years of treatments that he was eventually fitted with a three-chamber pacemaker defibrillator.

The mechanics of how this happened are complicated, and call for some speculation. But as far as Ernst is concerned, he believes his heart was beating so slowly that it was being run by its intrinsic rate, a slow, automatic heart rate generated within the heart. (The SA node normally fires an impulse between 60 and 100 beats per minute. Heart rates under this "intrinsic" or "built-in" rate are less coordinated.) The pacemaker paces the heart on demand. If Ernst's heart starts to beat below the set rate of the pacer (say 60 beats per minute), then the pacemaker delivers a stimulus.

The problem with some paced beats is that they aren't quite as good as our own. Because the pacing lead is attached to the right ventricular muscle, the signal starts in the RV, which contracts first, and then the signal arrives in the LV 100 milliseconds later, which contracts slightly later. Doctors refer to this sort of contraction as dyssynchronous. The dyssynchrony is less effective and, over time, can weaken the heart muscle in some cases.

You might think pacemakers sound awful. Who wants an asynchronous contraction? However, many patients do fine with a single pacing lead. And a paced beat is better than no heartbeat at all.

Ernst's three-lead system is called a cardiac resynchronization therapy (CRT) defibrillator. (Another name for it is biventricular pacing defibrillator.) It has pacing leads in the right and left ventricles, and those two leads pace the heart simultaneously — thus the heart contraction is synchronous and more effective.

Ernst compares his heart to an engine: "You don't want an engine idling too low; it will rock and jerk. Turn up the idle and it smooths out." His pacemaker keeps his ventricles coordinated. "They've got somebody monitoring your aortic output with a Doppler and the other guy is tuning the pacemaker, and he's trying to get the firing motor or the cylinders to get the maximum cardiac output for a given heart rate. I sort of have a dynamometer-tuned distributor."

Meanwhile, Ernst's cardiac output continues to slowly decline. He understands that the huge training volume he experienced in his life, that extreme overtraining, may have been a cause of the problem. "I think we can clearly conclude that if you're interested in health, you don't need to be doing these big volumes," he says now.

His resting heart rate keeps going up. His max heart rate continues to drop. And Ernst's humor keeps on ticking.

"I've got one line going down and the other going up," he says. "I guess when they cross, I'm dead."

9 | The takeaway

LENNARD ZINN, JOHN MANDROLA, AND CHRIS CASE

NOW THAT YOU'VE LEARNED about the many types of arrhythmias and the range of increased risks you place yourself under as an endurance athlete, it's crucial to understand how to improve your chances of staving off an irregular heartbeat. In this chapter, we'll look at heart rate monitors that can help you keep an eye on things, supplements that may help tamp down arrhythmia, and guidelines on what to do if you encounter someone having a heart attack or sudden cardiac arrest.

Monitors and diagnostic tools

Zinn was able to get diagnosis and treatment quickly because he was wearing a heart rate monitor (HRM). The first time he experienced atrial tachycardia, he had a record of it on his Garmin device, which was communicating with the monitor on his chest strap. He downloaded the graph and showed it to his cardiologist, which helped with his diagnosis.

Heart rate monitor

It is highly recommended that any athlete doing an intense workout or an extremely long workout wear a heart rate monitor. The most common type of HRM is a chest strap that communicates via Bluetooth to a wrist- or bike-mounted head unit. Self-contained wristwatch HRMs are also available, and Lazer offers bicycle helmets with a built-in optical heart-rate sensor that communicates remotely to any of a number of HRM units just as a chest monitor does.

When you select a monitor, get one that lets you download the data and review it later for irregularities. Generally, information from the HRM unit can be downloaded into databases like Garmin Express, Strava, and TrainingPeaks, and files can be e-mailed, which is convenient when your doctor asks to see the data you've collected.

As useful as a heart rate monitor can be, however, it's important to note that it will not be 100 percent accurate. To reduce erroneous readings, make sure the device has good contact with your skin. Try to correlate abnormal readings with abnormal sensations. Dr. Mandrola has seen many patients who thought they were having a problem with heart rate, but instead were simply seeing faulty readings from a monitor. This is not a knock on heart rate monitors; faulty tracings occur in the hospital too. In medicine, it's called an "artifact," and every time a doctor or nurse takes a board exam, one of the questions requires identification of an artifact.

AliveCor Kardia ECG

The AliveCor Kardia ECG consists of a smart-phone contact plate and an associated app. It's available for Apple and Android smartphones, tablet computers, and the Apple Watch, and it can be an extremely useful diagnostic tool for some athletes wondering about their hearts. It will catch arrhythmias only if the symptoms persist while sitting and relaxing, however.

If you are experiencing irregular heart rhythms, you may be able to use the device to answer many questions just by holding the two-contact unit, which sticks to the back of a smartphone or tablet computer, or sits adjacent to it. The user launches the Kardia app, clicks on "Record now," and touches two flat, rectangular electrodes with each hand while sitting quietly. A 30-second ECG tracing appears on the screen along with descriptions like "Normal," "Unreadable," or "Unclassified," or the device indicates an arrhythmia like atrial fibrillation. A cardiologist contracted by AliveCor performs the first reading remotely and gives a diagnosis within a couple of hours. Subsequent diagnoses are performed by computer, but the user can request an ECG review of any tracing done by the unit, either a "More Comprehensive" review for $19, or a "Quicker Response" review for $9.

The handheld AliveCor device can be useful in identifying the cause of rhythm problems. The first step in treating arrhythmia involves getting the right diagnosis, which often means recording the actual rhythm when it's happening. Before handheld devices like the Kardia came along, the only way to do this was with long-term monitors.

There are at least two drawbacks to the AliveCor Kardia. The first is that it won't work well during exercise. The second is its cost, which is not covered by insurance plans; on the other hand, it's only $99 (more if you get the blood-pressure add-on).

Holter monitor

If you are having symptoms you cannot figure out, especially while exercising, it's a good idea to request that your doctor prescribe a portable telemetric ECG device (a Holter monitor) for you. It often allows accurate diagnoses of electrical conditions in the heart that have not appeared on ECGs or stress tests in a doctor's office.

Supplements

Much research has looked at the efficacy of supplements in heart health. While some may help create a healthier heart and reduce your chances of developing an arrhythmia, others are effective in treating the symptoms of arrhythmias and their side effects. Let's look at the most popular and effective.

Coenzyme Q_{10}

Coenzyme Q_{10} (ubiquinone, and abbreviated to CoQ_{10}) is a coenzyme found in the cell mitochondria in most animals. It is required in aerobic respiration to produce energy in the form of ATP.

Numerous scientific studies have demonstrated that CoQ_{10} plays a key role in heart health, for reducing vascular disease, angina, cardiomyopathy, and arrhythmias.[1] Not only does CoQ_{10} tend to be low in patients with myocardial disease, but the lower the CoQ_{10}, the worse the symptoms. Additionally, nearly two-thirds of patients in severe heart failure showed subjective and objective improvement with a daily dose of 100 mg of CoQ_{10}.[2]

CoQ_{10} may be useful in treating arrhythmias, as some patients with premature ventricular contractions and no evidence of organic heart disease showed a reduction in PVCs after four to five weeks taking 60 mg/day of CoQ_{10}. The mean reduction in PVC frequency with CoQ_{10} supplementation was 85.7 percent in diabetics and considerably lower in other groups.[3]

Many pharmaceuticals, including tricyclic antidepressants, beta-blockers (prescribed to reduce heart arrhythmias and hypertension), and statins (prescribed to reduce cholesterol, treat coronary heart disease, and prevent stroke) can reduce blood CoQ_{10} levels. Even 14 days on atorvastatin causes a marked decrease in blood CoQ_{10} concentration.[4] Lovastatin also was shown to reduce blood CoQ_{10} concentration, and supplementing with CoQ_{10} improved cardiac function in patients taking lovastatin.[5] The most commonly reported adverse effect of statins relate to muscle pain or weakness, which could be explained by inhibition of CoQ_{10} synthesis.[6]

CoQ_{10} has also been shown in humans to stabilize cell membranes and to be a potent antioxidant (that is, an effective scavenger of free radicals, which are highly reactive due to unpaired valence electrons).[7] One human study reported that taking ubiquinol-10, the reduced form of CoQ_{10}, protected low-density lipoproteins (LDL, or "bad" cholesterol) more effectively from degradation due to oxidation by free radicals than did vitamin E.[8] Oxidation of LDL is now seen as a factor initiating the development of atherosclerosis, so CoQ_{10} may inhibit arterial blockage.

Meat and fish are the richest sources of dietary CoQ_{10}, followed by vegetable oils and avocados. Parsley, broccoli, grapes, and cauliflower are modest sources of CoQ_{10}.

Many approaches have been taken to improve the bioavailability of CoQ_{10} supplements, including micro- and nano-particles, oil suspension in soft-gel capsules, and water-soluble forms. Some CoQ_{10} sellers suggest taking the "trans-" form and not the "cis-" form of coenzyme Q_{10}, claiming that the body produces trans-CoQ_{10} ("trans" in the sense that its bonds to like groups are on opposite sides of the molecule), and that cis-CoQ_{10} (with bonds to like groups that are adjacent on the molecule) is a synthetic form not metabolized by the body. Others have suggested that the reduced "ubiquinol" form is more bioavailable. In any of its available forms, it appears to be safe to take, as no studies have shown an adverse effect to its ingestion at standard dosages.

L-carnitine

L-carnitine is an amino acid that transports fatty acids across the inner membrane into the mitochondria, where it is converted to energy. It also modulates the oxidation rate of fatty acids, transports waste products generated in the production of ATP out of the mitochondria, and participates in regulating cellular apoptosis (programmed cell death).

L-carnitine is available in supplements (and is naturally occurring in the body) as acetyl-L-carnitine (ALCAR), as L-carnitine fumarate, and as propionyl-L-carnitine.

According to a systematic review and meta-analysis of 13 controlled trials (N = 3,629), L-carnitine supplementation in the setting of a heart attack resulted in a 65 percent decrease in ventricular arrhythmias and a 40 percent reduction in the incidence of angina (chest discomfort caused by coronary artery disease).[9] Three issues with this trial limit its conclusions. First, each of the studies had wide confidence intervals, meaning the difference could have been due to chance. A second issue is that many of the included studies were not double-blinded. Third, the trials that drove the benefit seen in this review were performed in the 1990s, before heart attack care included stents.

Another study the same year attributed reductions and reversals of age-related mitochondrial damage to supplementation with acetyl-L-carnitine in rats.[10] That study also posits the effectiveness of L-carnitine in reducing arterial hypertension associated with vascular disease in humans.

These 2013 studies slightly supersede studies linking L-carnitine to a host of cardiovascular diseases.[11] The latter studies attribute plaque buildup in the arteries to high levels in the blood of a bacteria called TMAO. In the gut, L-carnitine is converted along with choline into a bacteria called TMA, which is then converted to TMAO in the liver. A 2011 study says that further study on L-carnitine is needed before recommending its supplementation for heart disorders.[12]

According to eminent biologist Dr. Bruce Ames from the University of California at Berkeley, free-radical production and mitochondrial decay are responsible for much of the aging process, and he proposes taking acetyl-L-carnitine to combat it along with a potent antioxidant, alpha-lipoic acid (ALA), to scavenge the free radicals produced by turning up the activity in aging mitochondria and to enhance the activity of other antioxidants like vitamins C and E, coenzyme Q_{10}, and glutathione.

L-carnitine is available in high concentrations in red meat. Fish, chicken, and milk are also sources of L-carnitine. Lower L-carnitine concentrations are found in some nuts, seeds, and legumes (sunflower, pumpkin, and sesame seeds; peanuts, beans, peas, and lentils), some vegetables (artichokes, asparagus, beet greens, broccoli, Brussels sprouts, collard greens, garlic, mustard greens, okra, parsley, kale), some fruits (apricots, bananas), and some grains (buckwheat, corn, millet, oatmeal, rice bran, rye, whole wheat, wheat bran, and wheat germ).

Iodine

Iodine is the heaviest element (atomic number 53) required for life by most living organisms. It is one of the halogens, which comprise the second-to-last column to the right on the periodic table of the elements; the other commonly occurring halogens—fluorine, chlorine, and bromine—are all lighter. Halogens are highly reactive and commonly combine with metals to form salts (hence the halogen name, which means "salt-producing").

The thyroid gland (located in the lower neck) requires iodine to produce the hormone thyroxine (T4; the number refers to the four iodine atoms in the molecule), which, after converting to the hormone triiodothyronine (T3), drives the metabolic functions of the body, of which blood circulation is primary. In addition to many of its other functions, the thyroid controls the body's metabolic rate, as well as the body's sensitivity to many hormones, some of which can also affect the heart's function.

As we discussed in Chapter 4, high levels of thyroid hormone cause AF, and addressing the thyroid problem with adequate bioavailability of iodine resolves the AF. Studies have linked iodine deficiency with hypertension,[13] and systolic blood pressure was found to be inversely related to urinary iodine excretion.

After the thyroid, the next highest iodine concentration is in breast tissue. The thyroid gland utilizes primarily iodide, while breast tissue utilizes iodine.[14] Iodine functions in the body as both an antioxidant and as an oxidant.

In an effort to prevent goiter and cretinism in the population, potassium iodide has been added in low concentrations to table salt since the 1920s. From a strictly dietary perspective, iodine tends to be low in people who eat no ocean fish or sea vegetables, little iodized salt, lots of breads and pastas (containing bromide), or follow a vegan or vegetarian diet (without sea vegetables).[15] In addition, since other halogens tend to bond to iodine receptors in the body, high environmental levels of other halogens block iodine uptake and exacerbate iodine deficiency.[16]

What are these halogens that can block iodine uptake? The halogens fluorine, chlorine, and bromine are increasingly common in the environment. In municipal water supplies, chlorine is added to kill bacteria, viruses, and protozoans, and fluoride is often added to prevent tooth decay. Bromine is added to flour as an anticaking agent and to pools and hot tubs as an antibacterial agent. It is a principal component of fire-retardant chemicals added to carpets, mattresses, and other furniture. Bromine is sprayed on crops and by pest exterminators as a fumigant to suffocate or poison insects, and it is an ingredient in a number of nasal sprays and inhalers. Perchlorate (one chlorine atom surrounded by four oxygens) is used in matches, fireworks, automotive air bags, rocket fuels, and in leather tanning, and it has become abundant in water, including ground water. The entire lower Colorado River has high perchlorate levels, and it not only supplies many southwestern cities and towns with water, but it also waters a large percentage of U.S. crops and livestock.

Like other halogens, iodine combines with metals (like potassium or sodium) to form salts, which increases its solubility in water. The standard iodine supplement, Lugol's solution, is 10 percent potassium iodide and 5 percent iodine. To properly utilize iodine, the body requires selenium to reduce the hydrogen peroxide with which the body oxidizes iodine. (The mitochondria produce hydrogen peroxide as a byproduct of the production of ATP, the body's energy source. Selenium is also required in the production of glutathione, a powerful antioxidant the body uses to eliminate free radicals, heavy metals, and chemical toxins.)[17]

One teaspoon of iodized salt contains approximately 400 µg (micrograms) of iodine. The Recommended Dietary Allowance (RDA) for iodine is as low as 90 µg/day for children (4–8 years) and as high as 290 µg/day for breast-feeding mothers in the United States and Canada.[18] By contrast, the average iodine intake in Japan is 1,000–3,000 µg/day (1–3 mg/day),[19] comes largely from seaweeds, and in some areas of the country is as high as 14 mg/day;[20] Japan has one of the world's lowest rates of coronary heart disease as well as a low rate of breast cancer.[21]

Because iodine is abundant in sea water, seaweed and seafood contain the most iodine, followed by meat and then eggs, dairy products, some vegetables, and, of course, iodized salt. The richest food sources of selenium are seafood and organ meats, followed by muscle meats, grains, and dairy products.[22] Iodine/iodide supplements are available in pill or liquid form.

Garlic

Garlic is a tasty and ubiquitous herb related to onions, leeks, and chives. The active chemical produced by the plant is allicin (from "allium," Latin for garlic), which also gives garlic its smell.

Garlic has traditionally been used to treat high or low blood pressure, high cholesterol (either inherited or not), coronary heart disease, heart attack, atherosclerosis, and reduced blood flow due to narrowed arteries.[23]

A hydrophobic chemical, allicin can pass through a cell membrane's lipid bilayer without damaging it. Cells can rapidly metabolize it to access its cardio-protective effects. These include reducing the tension in blood vessel walls (vasorelaxation) and alleviating some cardiovascular disease conditions, including cardiac hypertrophy, hyperlipidemia, hyperglycemia, angiogenesis, and platelet aggregation. Allicin also acts as an antioxidant to protect the cardiovascular system by scavenging reactive oxygen species; these highly reactive molecules include free radicals, peroxides, lipid peroxides, and heavy metals. It also stimulates production of the body's most powerful antioxidant, glutathione.[24]

If you aren't a fan of garlic in its most common form, it is also available as a supplement. Some garlic supplements have an "enteric" coating to protect them from stomach acids so that they will instead dissolve in the intestine.

Magnesium

Magnesium plays a critical role in a host of physiological functions: It activates enzymes, contributes to energy production, and helps regulate levels of calcium, copper, zinc, potassium, vitamin D, and other important nutrients in the body. Your cells need a steady supply of magnesium to maintain proper smooth muscle function in your blood vessels. In addition, magnesium can help your body shuttle potassium and sodium, two other essential electrolytes, into and out of cells, maintaining proper balance (homeostasis).

Unfortunately, many people are seriously low in this mineral. Shortages of magnesium can be caused by a number of factors, including prolonged stress, certain pharmaceuticals such as diuretics, diet (including drinking too much coffee, soda, or alcohol, or eating too much salt), heavy menstrual periods, and excessive sweating.

Magnesium deficiencies can lead to muscle weakness and spasms as well as a host of cardiovascular problems, including congestive heart failure, atherosclerosis, chest pain (coronary vasospasm), high blood pressure, cardiac arrhythmias, cardiomyopathy, heart attack, and sudden cardiac death.

Indeed, proper levels of magnesium are essential to heart health. Studies suggest a possible association between a modestly lower risk of coronary heart disease in men and increased magnesium intake. In one study of women, higher dietary intake of magnesium was associated with a lower risk of sudden cardiac death.[25] Magnesium helps maintain a normal heart rhythm, and doctors sometimes administer it intravenously to reduce the chance of atrial fibrillation and cardiac arrhythmia.

Since it plays such an important role in so many physiological functions, a ready supply of magnesium in an athletic diet is vital. Natural sources include whole grains, fish and seafood, leafy green vegetables, soy products, brown rice, bananas, apricots, seeds, and nuts. The foods highest in magnesium include kelp, tofu, figs, and pumpkin seeds.

If you have a diet that is not adequate in magnesium, you might consider an "insurance" dose of magnesium from a high-quality multivitamin or mineral supplement. Look for easily absorbable forms such as magnesium orotate or magnesium citrate. Remember, magnesium works in concert with other nutrients, particularly B vitamins, CoQ_{10}, and vitamin E. Furthermore, magnesium and calcium work together at very precise ratios to ensure your heart functions properly. Talk to your doctor before taking magnesium supplements if you have a history of cardiac or kidney issues.

Aspirin

For more than 100 years, aspirin has been used as a pain reliever. Since the 1970s, aspirin has also been used to prevent and manage heart disease and stroke. New guidelines from the US Preventive Services Task Force, an independent panel of national experts in prevention and evidence-based medicine, recommend that adults 50 to 59 years old who have a 10 percent or greater risk of cardiovascular disease, are not at an increased risk for bleeding, and have a life expectancy of at least 10 years take a low-dose aspirin daily to prevent cardiovascular disease and colorectal cancer.

Aspirin lowers the risk of cardiovascular disease through its ability to decrease inflammation, which is a component of plaque buildup. (Inflamed plaque is more likely to cause a heart attack or stroke.) Aspirin fights inflammation by blocking the action of an enzyme called cyclooxygenase. When this enzyme is blocked, the body is less able to produce prostaglandins, chemicals that facilitate the inflammatory response.

Prostaglandins are also involved in triggering clotting. Thus, aspirin's other effects on your heart pertain more to its ability to prevent clots than to affect arrhythmias specifically. Indeed, in some studies the use of aspirin has been shown to reduce the risk of stroke or systemic embolism in AF patients.

However, the medical community is not in agreement on the use of aspirin. Some argue there is no compelling evidence that aspirin reduces the risk of stroke in patients with AF. In fact, European guidelines recommend against aspirin use for stroke prevention for AF. American guidelines give aspirin a halfhearted endorsement, saying it may reduce the risk of stroke, but much less so than clot-blocking drugs.

In people without arrhythmia issues, the benefit of aspirin for prevention of strokes and heart attacks depends on the underlying risk of the patient. At the high-risk end, patients with cardiac stents, those who have had prior strokes due to blockages, smokers, or those with cardiac risk factors such as diabetes, high blood pressure, and elevated cholesterol tend to benefit from aspirin. Here, the benefit from the clot-inhibiting property of aspirin outweighs the harm it can cause by increasing one's risk of bleeding. However, younger people without these high-risk conditions have such a low rate of cardiac events that the negative attributes of aspirin outweigh any small benefit.

Hawthorn

Hawthorn (Crataegus species) has been used to treat heart disease since the first century. By the early 1800s, American doctors were using it to treat circulatory disorders and respiratory illnesses. Traditionally, the berries of this thorny shrub of the rose family were used to treat heart problems ranging from irregular heartbeat to high blood pressure, chest pain (angina), hardening of the arteries, and heart failure. Today, the leaves and flowers are used medicinally, although their mechanism is not clear.

Still, there is growing evidence of its usefulness. Several studies have recognized anti-arrhythmic properties of hawthorn. Others suggest it can help to protect against heart disease and help control high blood pressure and high cholesterol. Both animal and human studies suggest hawthorn increases coronary artery blood flow, improves circulation, and lowers blood pressure.[26]

Animal and laboratory studies report that hawthorn contains antioxidants, including oligomeric procyandins (also found in grapes) and quercetin. These compounds may help stop some of the damage from free radicals, especially when it comes to heart disease.

It is important to note that while the use of herbs is a time-honored approach to treating disease, you should never self-treat heart conditions without telling your doctor, and should only use hawthorn under your doctor's supervision. Herbs can contain components that may trigger side effects and interact with other herbs, supplements, or medications.[27]

If you are currently being treated with any of the following medications, you should not use hawthorn without first talking to your provider:

- Digoxin: Hawthorn may enhance the activity of digoxin, a
  medication used for irregular heart rhythms.

- Beta-blockers: These drugs are used to treat heart disease by lowering blood pressure and dilating blood vessels. Hawthorn can make the effects of these drugs stronger. They include atenolol (Tenormin), metoprolol (Lopressor, Toprol-XL), and propranolol (Inderal, Inderal LA).

- Calcium channel blockers: These drugs are used to treat high blood pressure and angina by dilating blood vessels. Hawthorn can strengthen the effects of these drugs. They include amlopidine (Norvasc), diltiazem (Cardizem), and nifedipine (Procardia).

Drug cautions

Nonsteroidal anti-inflammatory drugs (NSAIDs) inhibit a class of enzymes in the inflammatory response called cyclooxygenases, which decrease the production of prostaglandins (chemicals that lead to the pain, redness, and swelling of inflammation). NSAIDs are primarily sold over the counter—ibuprofen and naproxen, for example—and are also available by prescription in drugs such as diclofenac or celecoxib. Nearly everyone has felt the pain-relief effect of NSAIDs; the drugs work pretty well.

The downside is that prostaglandins also play an important role in protecting the lining of the stomach and modulating kidney and blood platelet (clotting) function. That's a pretty big downside, especially for athletes.

NSAID harm to major organ systems

NSAIDs disrupt the normal protective processes of the stomach and small intestine. Couple this adverse effect with their aspirin-like effect in the blood and it's no wonder that they increase the risk of bleeding from the gut.

NSAIDs also have major effects on the kidney. To oversimplify somewhat, think of the kidney as a big filter. Blood flows through the filter and comes out cleansed. A major determinant of how well a filter functions is the rate of flow through the filter. NSAIDs decrease the flow of blood through the kidney, thereby decreasing its filtering ability. This effect is magnified in the presence of dehydration (athletes pay heed), other medicines, high blood pressure, and diabetes. What's more, NSAIDs can also have an allergic-like effect on the kidney, an effect called interstitial nephritis. It's unpredictable and in some cases irreversible, which can lead to dialysis.

Numerous observational studies have suggested an association between long-term use of NSAIDs and adverse cardiovascular outcomes.[28] Most of these studies suggest people with known heart disease are at highest risk of NSAID-induced events such as stroke, heart attack, and arrhythmia. The likely way these drugs affect the heart and blood vessels is by increasing blood pressure and altering platelet stickiness.

Could the drugs lead to atrial fibrillation? One study, from Denmark, looked at more than 32,000 patients who were seen for new-onset atrial fibrillation.[29] Researchers compared these patients to a control group of patients matched for similar medical characteristics. Use of NSAIDs increased the odds of having AF by 17 to 27 percent. And the association was strongest for new users. More recently, another group of Danish authors confirmed the association of NSAID use and AF in a 13-year study of more than 8,000 older (average age 68 years) participants.[30]

NSAIDs have long been marketed as better and safer pain relievers than alternatives like acetaminophen, but the data here are dubious. A study in the *New England Journal of Medicine,* from a group of researchers at Indiana University, showed that acetaminophen and ibuprofen performed equally well for the relief of arthritic knee pain.[31]

A major drawback to these supposedly "anti-inflammatory" drugs is that they may aggravate intestinal inflammation during and after exercise. Researchers from the Netherlands set out to test the safety of the drugs when used as pre-exercise pain relievers. In a controlled study using nine cyclists, the researchers found that both ibuprofen consumption alone and cycling alone induced slight intestinal injury as measured by leak of a gut protein (similar to troponin leak from heart muscle). The kicker was that cycling while on ibuprofen aggravated intestinal injury and induced gut barrier dysfunction in normal people. In other words, these cyclists leaked poop from their bowel into the body.[32]

Should you avoid NSAIDs for pain relief altogether? Small doses, taken occasionally, may help minor aches or pains. The problem comes when the drugs are taken regularly, or in high doses, or in combination with intense exercise. As with so many of the topics in this book, moderation is key.

Decongestant and "cold" tablets

Over-the-counter medications labeled as decongestants usually include the drug pseudoephedrine. This drug works by stimulating adrenaline receptors in the nasal and bronchial passages, which helps relieve clogged airways during an illness. The problem is the drugs don't just stimulate adrenaline receptors in the nose and lungs; they also cause total-body stimulation of adrenaline. This can lead to high blood pressure and arrhythmias. In patients who are susceptible to heart disease, or have heart disease or even benign arrhythmias like PACs or PVCs, the stimulant drugs can worsen symptoms. One trick clever doctors use in treating patients with arrhythmias is to get them off decongestants; the symptoms often resolve.

Note that there is a difference between antihistamine (allergy) medications and decongestants. Allergy medications, such as cetirizine (Zyrtec), fexofenadine (Allegra), loratadine (Claritin), and diphenhydramine (Benadryl) do not have stimulant properties and are therefore much less likely to cause or exacerbate heart issues. Be careful, though; these drugs are sometimes combined with pseudoephedrine, as in Allegra-D, where the "D" indicates the decongestant.

What to do if someone has a heart attack or sudden cardiac arrest

Though people often use the terms "heart attack" and "sudden cardiac arrest" interchangeably, they are not synonyms. A heart attack occurs when blood flow to the heart muscle cells is blocked; sudden cardiac arrest (SCA) occurs when the heart malfunctions and suddenly stops beating unexpectedly. In simple terms, a heart attack is a circulation problem, and sudden cardiac arrest is an electrical problem.

A heart attack occurs when a blocked artery prevents oxygen-rich blood from reaching a section of the heart. If the blocked artery is not reopened quickly, the part of the heart normally nourished by that artery begins to die. The longer a person goes without treatment, the greater the damage. Symptoms of a heart attack may be immediate and intense. More often, however, symptoms start slowly and persist for hours, days, or weeks before a heart attack. Unlike with sudden cardiac arrest, the heart usually does not stop beating during a heart attack. It's also important to note that the symptoms of heart attack can be different in men and women.

Sudden cardiac arrest can occur without warning. It is triggered by an electrical malfunction in the heart that causes an arrhythmia. With its pumping action disrupted, the heart cannot pump blood to the brain, lungs, or other organs. Seconds later, a person loses consciousness and a pulse. Death occurs within minutes if the victim does not receive treatment. But if treated within those crucial first few minutes, the condition is reversible in most victims. Survival chances are increased if victims of SCA are treated before emergency personnel arrive at the scene.

Though the two conditions are not the same, there are some links between them. Sudden cardiac arrest can occur after a heart attack, or during recovery. Heart attacks increase the risk for sudden cardiac arrest, though most heart attacks do not lead to arrest. As you now know, other heart conditions may also disrupt the heart's rhythm and lead to sudden cardiac arrest. These include a thickened heart muscle (hypertrophic cardiomyopathy), heart failure, and Long QT syndrome.

In both heart attack and sudden cardiac arrest, fast action can often mean the difference between life and death. According to the American Heart Association, over 320,000 out-of-hospital cardiac arrests occur annually in the United States. That's more than breast cancer, prostate cancer, colorectal cancer, AIDS, traffic accidents, house fires, and gunshot wounds combined. Only 11 percent survive, according to the Sudden Cardiac Arrest Foundation.

What to do: heart attack

The American Heart Association recommends that even if you're not sure it's a heart attack, call 9-1-1 or your emergency response number. Every minute matters. Emergency medical services staff can begin treatment when they arrive at the scene, which will often be sooner than if someone travels to the hospital by private car. EMS staff are also trained to revive someone whose heart has stopped. Patients with chest pain who arrive by ambulance usually receive faster treatment at the hospital, too.

What to do: sudden cardiac arrest

The following steps are recommended by the Sudden Cardiac Arrest Foundation:

- Learn how to recognize sudden cardiac arrest. When someone is in SCA, he or she suddenly loses consciousness, stops breathing normally, and exhibits no signs of life.

- Decide to help. Victims of SCA can only be saved if bystanders intervene immediately. There may not be enough time to wait for professional medical personnel to arrive at the scene. The chances for survival decrease by 10 percent with each passing

minute after collapse. You may be the victim's only hope
for survival.

- Call 9-1-1. Or, if you are with someone or can get help nearby,
  have that person call 9-1-1 while you start treatment. Be sure
  to communicate with a specific person—"John, call 9-1-1";
  otherwise, bystanders in a crowd may hesitate and wait for
  someone else to help.

- If an automated external defibrillator (AED) is immediately
  available, grab it or send someone to retrieve it and bring it to
  you. Apply the AED electrode pads to the person's chest as shown
  on diagrams that accompany the AED. Follow the voice and
  visual prompts. If a person is in a heart rhythm that warrants a
  shock, the AED will automatically shock the heart. This electrical
  therapy can restore a normal heart rhythm if it is used quickly
  enough. Do not be concerned with harming the victim. AEDs
  are safe and effective and can only help. AEDs will not shock
  someone who does not need to be shocked. Emergency medical
  dispatchers can provide additional guidance.

- If an AED is not immediately available and you are trained in
  CPR, begin compressions.

- If an AED is not immediately available and you are not trained in
  CPR, push down hard and fast in the center of the chest (2-inch
  depth, 100 pumps/minute). Continue.

Bystander intervention in medical emergencies

Research indicates that bystander action in medical emergencies is complex. Several factors affect whether a bystander is more or less likely to act. Factors that decrease likelihood of bystander intervention include

- Public location: Compared to health care professionals, laypersons are significantly less likely to offer help in emergencies that occur in public places.

- Ignorance and confusion: When people do not understand what is happening or are confused about the unfolding situation, they are less likely to intervene.

- Difficulty in recognizing medical emergencies: It is difficult to perceive that a medical emergency is occurring because indications often are ambiguous. Consequently, bystanders often delay in deciding to call EMS for help.

- Lack of confidence and competence: A person who does not feel competent to deal with an emergency is unlikely to offer even minimal help. CPR is difficult to learn, and CPR skill retention is poor when these skills are not used regularly.

- Presence of other bystanders: The presence of others leads to a diminished sense of personal responsibility.

- Unpleasant physical characteristics: Regurgitation, blood, dentures, and other characteristics of the victim encountered during rescue breathing tend to dissuade bystanders from intervening.

- Fear of harming the patient: A lack of knowledge and skills inhibit CPR use among families of high-risk patients.

- Fear of using AEDs incorrectly: People unfamiliar with AEDs tend to be fearful of using them incorrectly.

Factors that increase the likelihood of bystander intervention include

- Size of the community in which the bystander lives or grew up: Individuals who grew up in rural areas are more likely to help than individuals from urban areas. People from non-metropolitan areas are more likely to help than their counterparts.

- Presence at the time of the event: Bystanders who witness the emergency are more likely to help than those who arrive after the emergency has occurred.

- Previous emergency training and positions of responsibility: People with CPR training or other emergency training and people with positions of responsibility in their organizations are more likely to help in SCA.

- Availability of AED: When AEDs are available, bystanders are more likely to initiate CPR.

Implantable cardioverter defibrillator therapy

Individuals considered at definite high risk for sudden cardiac arrest, like Mike Endicott (Chapter 4) and Paul Ernst (Chapter 8), can undergo implantable cardioverter defibrillator therapy. An ICD is a small, computerized device that is implanted in the upper chest of patients who are at risk for sudden cardiac arrest. Most ICDs would fit easily in the palm of the hand. The ICD detects abnormal heart rhythms, delivers electrical energy to the heart muscle, and restores a normal heartbeat.

While pacemakers are designed to speed up a slow heart rate, ICDs are designed to slow down a fast heartbeat. All ICDs also have built-in pacemakers and can address both problems. The ICD has two parts: the lead(s), which monitor the heart rhythm and deliver energy, and the generator, which houses a battery and small computer. Energy is stored in the battery until it is needed. When it is not needed, the ICD simply monitors the heart rhythm.

ICDs are programmed to address the specific needs of each patient. They may be programmed to address one or more of the following problems to restore a normal heartbeat:

- Anti-tachycardia pacing: Delivery of small electrical impulses when the heart is beating too fast.

- Cardioversion: Delivery of a low-energy shock to convert an arrhythmia back to sinus rhythm.

- Defibrillation: Delivery of a high-energy shock when the heart is beating dangerously fast (ventricular fibrillation).

- Bradycardia pacing: Delivery of small electrical impulses when the heart is beating too slowly.

A patient may or may not be aware when the ICD detects an abnormal rhythm and restores a normal rhythm. Patients usually do not feel small impulses. However, cardioversion may feel like a thump on the chest. Defibrillation may feel like a kick in the chest, or the patient may become unconscious and not feel the shock. If a shock is delivered, the patient should

- Sit or lie down.

- Call 9-1-1 if he or she does not feel well.

- Call the doctor within 24 hours if he or she does feel well.

Getting an ICD is a major decision because the device comes with some risks. These include surgical risks of the implant (approximately 1–2 percent of all cases), inappropriate shocks (shocks for non-life-threatening rhythms), late infection (rare), lead malfunction, hardware recalls (rare), and anxiety and depression after a shock. The device battery lasts between 5 and 8 years, and if the heart condition remains, most patients have another surgery to replace the device. Generator change, as it is called, can be done without admission to the hospital, but it carries a slightly higher risk of complication than the original implant. Patients with ICDs can return to physical activity. And the results of a recent multinational registry study suggest many athletes with ICDs can engage in vigorous and competitive sports without physical injury or failure to terminate the arrhythmia despite the occurrence of both inappropriate and appropriate shocks.[33]

CASE STUDY

Jason Agosta: Highly symptomatic paroxysmal atrial fibrillation

Diagnosed at age 49

CHRIS CASE

JASON AGOSTA started running when he was 15. In his prime, he was an elite distance runner, specializing in the 5,000-meter, 10,000-meter, and cross-country events.

He represented Australia at two world championships, one in cross-country and the other at the 5-kilometer distance. He was unsuccessful at making the Olympic team despite intense effort.

"Between the ages of 18 and 25, trying to make that Olympic team, training was absolutely all consuming, and I had no real guidance on my development as an athlete," he says. During his peak years, he would regularly complete two to three intense sessions a week and one long, harder run. His total mileage was typically 60–70 miles per week.

"At 5 and 10K, training is intense endurance, and certainly more intense than the guys I ran with who were doing marathons," Agosta says.

By age 30, he had retired. He continued to run, although it was most always at an easier pace and with much less volume.

In late 2014, at the age of 47, Agosta began to experience skipping and fluttering in his heart, without consistency. Family and work stresses continued to build into the middle of 2015 when the arrhythmia became more consistent and his level of fatigue began to rise.

"At their worst, I was having outrageous palpitations and fatigue," he says.

Finally, in July 2015, he had to stop during a trail run. He knew something wasn't right—his heart rate and breathing were wildly out-of-sync.

Less than two weeks later, he had a stress echocardiogram and, as he puts it, "blew up totally."

"I couldn't believe it as I was really fit and strong still. And I wasn't overdoing the exercise. But I was aware of the degenerative changes acquired through running," he says.

His physician, Dr. André La Gerche, the head of the sports cardiology and cardiac magnetic resonance imaging group at the Baker IDI Heart and Diabetes Institute in Melbourne, Australia, prescribed the anti-arrhythmic drug sotalol in September 2015.

"The issue with athletes is that they often find sotalol to be intolerable," La Gerche says. "In many it reduces their exercise capacity, makes them feel like a 'diesel engine' and can cause a more general fatigue. However, like in Jason's case, I also find that some athletes tolerate it very well and that it is very effective at preventing frequent bouts of AF."

La Gerche notes that all AF drugs have their issues. For instance, Flecainide can convert atrial fibrillation to flutter and enable the heart to conduct at very fast rates, an uncommon but potentially very serious problem, he says. Another anti-arrhythmic drug, amiodarone, has a huge list of serious side effects that become common if the drug is used long-term, according to La Gerche.

"Many people say that it is not worth trying sotalol in athletes because they never tolerate it. This is not my experience," La Gerche says. "Although they may be a minority, some athletes do extremely well on this drug and I will continue to try it."

Agosta's treatment experience with sotalol, for one, has been extremely positive.

"Things have been ideal since I started taking it," Agosta says. "Only three times in 12 months have I had to take three tablets rather than the usual two in a day."

And he continues to exercise. He rides his mountain bike, and often intensely without issue. "I can bike really well now with no trouble. Three-hour endurance rides are no hassle," he says. He also does strength training with no worries.

"I've stopped running since July 2015, which seems unusual to many people. But for me it just doesn't feel 'right' anymore," Agosta says. "I'm not sure why and I can't explain it. But I'm not troubled at all by it."

Agosta has no doubt that his many years of elite training have contributed to his arrhythmia. He admits to being addicted to running when he was in his prime. That wasn't the case through his 30s and 40s, and now he makes sure to minimize stress at both home and work.

Unfortunately, even if a patient's initial response to an anti-arrhythmic drug is good, the majority of patients tend to regress, according to La Gerche. However, there is great variability between patients: Some will stabilize and remain symptom free for many years, others won't.

Agosta is one of the fortunate.

"Sotalol has saved me," he says.

Epilogue

CHRIS CASE

THE SUN IS STILL SHINING BRIGHT on the Flatirons above Boulder. It is yet another perfect day in an outdoors paradise. And Lennard Zinn is again pedaling his bike to the top of Flagstaff Mountain, albeit at a much gentler pace. He will never again make a Strava KOM attempt on this or any other mountain road.

He's comfortable with that state of affairs—now. It took him years to accept it. But his wake-up call at the age of 55 is one he's ultimately glad to have received. It will allow him to lead a longer, healthier life, filled with more bike rides, ski runs, and paddle strokes than he would have had under his old regimen, in which he was always pushing, pushing, pushing. And, more importantly, he is simply happier.

Like thousands of other athletes who have come to terms with their own similar situations, Zinn has found that there is indeed life after athletic competition. He would be the first to tell you it can be a long process to recognize that truth. He'd also understand if, even after reading this book, you still had the urge to keep chasing results that only other masters competitors would ever care about. He had that same attitude for a while.

The evidence we've presented in *The Haywire Heart* can be alarming. If you are a committed endurance athlete, you will probably need to recalibrate your understanding of medicine and exercise to accept the fact that what you once thought was the very best thing for your health can turn out to be the exact opposite, if taken to the extreme.

The evidence for this continues to accumulate. Research has been difficult to conduct because of the limited number of people who make up the endurance-athlete population, but piles of data from epidemiologic, observational, and animal studies already exist. They cannot be ignored.

An athlete's heart is repeatedly put under unusual strain—mechanically, physiologically, electrically. Years of endurance training inevitably cause inflammation, scarring, and stretching. These changes to the fundamental structure of the heart can irrevocably alter how it operates. In the specific case of atrial fibrillation, when these findings are placed in the broader context of observational studies on common lifestyle stresses that also cause inflammation and stretching, it becomes easier to see how long-term endurance exercise probably leads to AF. The fact that detraining often fixes the problem only bolsters that hypothesis.

Likewise, compelling evidence from both "marathon rats" and individuals with arrhythmogenic right ventricular cardiomyopathy suggests that endurance exercise can promote severe disease in the right ventricle. This evidence is further reinforced by observational and mechanistic studies that have looked at biomarkers of heart damage in endurance athletes, as well as imaging studies that revealed consistent dilation and power loss in the right ventricle. Given the nature of these studies, the findings aren't conclusive, but they suggest a high plausibility of correlation between endurance exercise and disease.

It's important to note, too, that athletes who begin their endurance lifestyle in middle age come to it with accumulated wear, tear, and neglect from their younger years. There's no doubt that it's good to get fit at any age, but atherosclerosis is a disease that slowly builds. A past history of unhealthy habits may not be nullified by a new habit of running, skiing, or cycling.

Most athletes can't help but push themselves really hard fairly often. But as we age, especially into our 50s and 60s, we need more rest after hard exertion. While it seems obvious that recovery time would increase with age, the physiological causes are not fully understood. According to a 2008 report in the *Journal of Aging and Physical Activity,* one of the most credible explanations is that aging muscles are more susceptible to exercise-induced damage and are slower to adapt and repair.[1]

When we combine this finding with the anecdotal observation that busy people rarely devote enough time to resting, it's easy to see how the strain of training and life can rise to an unhealthy level. So why doesn't every endurance athlete develop an arrhythmia?

It's a bit like the story with cigarette smokers. Not all of them get cancer or heart disease; some pick up the habit and still manage to wheeze into old age. But most don't.

It is clear that many athletes—probably most—do not develop heart disease or arrhythmias. But some do. Why these afflictions strike some and not others is still unknown. But what is known from the aforementioned studies is that overdosing on exercise can increase your risk of suffering serious consequences that in many cases necessitate life-altering changes, sometimes to avoid the potential for tragedy.

The message, therefore, seems to be that it would be wise to take a personal inventory of your training load and slow down before you reach that breaking point. When you train hard, rest just as hard. More rest may add years to your training life as well as to your actual life. (There's a good chance it'll make you faster too.)

As you surely noticed, the missing component in all of the athletic case histories we included in this book was rest. This is not a case of selection bias on the part of the authors; it's a foundational component of the incidence of arrhythmia in the athlete's heart.

If you're like the athletes profiled in this book, decades of training likely will have precipitated the abnormal substrate for arrhythmia described in Chapter 3. Your years of training and competition have made you more susceptible to the development of an arrhythmia because of the underlying inflammation, scarring, and atrial enlargement of your heart.

The complexity of the heart's physiology, human genetics, and a person's lifestyle and stress level make it difficult to predict when and in which heart something will malfunction, or whether a catastrophic event will take place. In every individual, years of cumulative variables would need to be considered to fully understand what went wrong or which threshold was breached on a particular day. Small insults to the heart—

easily dismissed as benign or random events—might be accruing in the background. Epic endurance events and the many hours of training that precede them keep piling up. Add to that cocktail a stressful lifestyle or a traumatic life event, for example, and an abstract watercolor of billowing clouds building on the distant horizon begins to appear. You probably won't make out the storm if you aren't looking for it. Add another stressful event, however, or maybe just a common cold, and one day that watercolor quickly becomes a high-definition feature film on arrhythmia. You've been struck.

That doesn't have to be the case. Have you ever felt that flutter in your chest? Ever thought, *That's odd. What was that?* Maybe you dismissed it. *I couldn't possibly have something wrong with my heart. I'm an athlete. I'm fit. I'm invincible.* You wouldn't be the first to disregard that subtle blip of warning.

But how much is too much? Where is that line? If you have an arrhythmia, you've likely already crossed it. For the rest of us, it's not as easy to know. We might be familiar with that pesky feeling of too little exercise, that we've got to get out right now, but there's great uncertainty about what is too much and what might send a person over the edge.

If the hints are there for you, pay attention. If you are still pushing yourself as hard as you were 10 years ago, it may be time to check in with a doctor. If you've felt a racing heart, chest pressure or pain, or labored breathing that seems to come too soon, or if you have fainted or just can't rebound the way you used to, a checkup could answer many questions. You may walk out with some good advice from an expert. It may help you reduce your risk of developing a haywire heart. It may save your life.

If instead you are one of the unfortunate individuals who has already developed an arrhythmia, your athletic life is not necessarily over. As you learned from the case studies in this book, passionate athletes find ways to live fulfilling lives after their diagnosis. Initially, you may not think so. You may pass through stages of anger, denial, fear. You may feel guilt, or ask yourself if you caused these issues by constantly striving for more. But if you are well-informed, persistent, and patient, a rich life awaits.

This book is the most comprehensive guide to the subject of endurance sports and heart health. It is filled with sound, practical advice. But it isn't meant to frighten you into becoming a full-time spectator. We present the information as it is known at this time. What you do with it is up to you, though we certainly encourage caution and thoughtfulness.

From a medical standpoint, the evidence here is critical for doctors to digest and understand. As more people pursue endurance sports, physicians will see more arrhythmias related to those demanding athletic challenges. Successful treatment of heart disorders, like all medical therapies, begins with a foundation of knowledge and an understanding of how to apply it to patients on an individual basis. When patients and doctors have all the available information, the odds of positive outcomes increases.

ACKNOWLEDGMENTS

Chris Case. I must first thank my incredible wife, Jessica, and our adorable daughter, Anika, for being exceedingly patient and supportive during the writing of this book. Without them by my side every step of the way, this book (or at least my portion) would not exist.

It should go without saying that each of the individuals whom I interviewed in the writing of the case studies—Gene Kay, Genevieve Halvorsen, Mark Taylor, Dave Scott, Paul Ernst, Jenni Lutze, Jason Agosta, and Mike Endicott—deserves my deepest gratitude for sharing his or her story. Their willingness to bare the depth and breadth of their journeys has made *The Haywire Heart* much more than just a story of heart disease. Their appreciation of that impact on people's understanding of the connection between endurance sports and heart health is to be commended.

There were others who shared their life-changing diagnoses but whose stories did not make it into the book: Andy Paulin, Greg Welch, and Doug Smith deserve grateful thanks for sharing their tales.

Doctors André La Gerche and Adrian Elliott were invaluable in helping me connect with athletes afflicted with arrhythmias. Their enthusiasm for explaining their patients' histories enriched the message of each case study.

Both in their generous personal conversations with me and through their research and writing, Doctors Mark Griffiths and Duncan Simpson contributed to my understanding of behavioral addictions, and specifically exercise addiction.

Trevor Connor provided critical feedback that resulted in a more nuanced understanding of human physiology and heart function.

I must recognize coauthor Lennard Zinn for sharing the tale of his first arrhythmic event with me. It was the impetus that led to the initial article in *VeloNews* and, ultimately, to this book.

John Mandrola. New writers require lots of help. I thank my wife and best friend, Dr. Staci Mandrola, for her support (and vocabulary help) over our 26 years together. My daughter, Catherine, and son, Will, grinned when they learned that their dad had become a blogger. Thanks to them for keeping me grounded.

Conversations with my friends and cycling mates Robert Bobrow, John May, Bob Dantoni, and Curtis Tolson helped formulate many of my views on athletics—and all things obvious.

Larry Creswell, a heart surgeon, triathlete, and publisher of the Athlete's Heart Blog (www.athletesheart.org), has been generous with his time and review of our manuscript. His commonsense interpretation of sports science and clear writing are worth your time.

The day that Shelley Wood, now an editor with TCTMD.com, then the news director of theHeart.org | Medscape Cardiology (www.medscape.com/cardiology), called to offer me a job as a physician writer changed my life. Thank you, Shelley. Over the past years, the editorial and journalist team at Medscape patiently nurtured me into the world of editorial writing. They are true pros. Special thanks to my current editor at Medscape, Tricia Ward. It's crazy how much a good editor helps a writer.

I also thank sports scientist Adrian Elliott in Adelaide, Australia, and electrophysiology colleague Andreas Müssigbrodt in Leipzig, Germany, for many spirited conversations about science and sports. Someday Andreas and I *will* have a scientific paper published together.

Finally, to my coauthors, Chris and Lennard, and VeloPress, I am grateful for including me in this project. It's been fun.

Lennard Zinn. This book never would have happened if I hadn't developed a heart arrhythmia, so that rightfully should be acknowledged first. And when it happened, I want to thank Doctors Shannon Sovndal, Jamie Doucet, Robert Rea, and Sameer Oza for their care and for persevering in communicating the reality of my condition through my denial of it. Above all, I want to thank my wife, Sonny, and my good friend Dag Selander for staying the night in the hospital with me and—along with my daughters, Emily and Sarah—for always supporting me before and since.

When my wife was pregnant 30 years ago, it seemed as though women all around us were pregnant, whereas I hadn't noticed very many pregnant people before. It was much the same with heart arrhythmia. After I was diagnosed with one, I suddenly seemed to be surrounded by fellow athletes with similar heart conditions. Almost universally, those friends who had dealt with cardiac arrhythmia were supportive and encouraging. Many of them became resources I continue to rely on. I want to thank all of them, specifically Mike Endicott, Gene and Clint Kay, and Mike and Karen Hogan, for their continual support.

For their assistance in my understanding of the issues and for their support, I thank Doctors Carl Reynolds, Pete Watson, Craig Pearson, Charley Cropley, Bill Campbell, Henry Walker, William Sauer, and Duy Nguyen. Thanks also to John Thompson, Mark Stewart, Clark ("Corky") Grimm, Bruce Gabow, Peter Marshall, Tom Knox, Paul Fuller, Heidi Dohse, and Jivan West for filling out my knowledge base. And, above all, thanks to Chris Case and John Mandrola for writing this book with me. Your tireless efforts, fantastic research, and wonderful writing make this a book of which I'm extremely proud.

Collectively, the authors would like to thank the staff of VeloPress, specifically publisher and editor Ted Costantino, who pushed the idea on them in the first place (along with a breakneck schedule), and managing editor Connie Oehring and creative director Vicki Hopewell for their many contributions to the final work.

NOTES

Introduction

1. R. K. Pathak et al., "Impact of CARDIOrespiratory FITness on Arrhythmia Recurrence in Obese Individuals with Atrial Fibrillation: The CARDIO-FIT Study," *Journal of American College of Cardiology* 66, no. 9 (2015): 985–996.

2. S. N. Blair et al., "Physical Fitness and All-Cause Mortality: A Prospective Study of Healthy Men and Women," *Journal of the American Medical Association* 262, no. 17 (1989): 2395–2401.

3. C. P. Wen et al., "Minimum Amount of Physical Activity for Reduced Mortality and Extended Life Expectancy: A Prospective Cohort Study," *Lancet* 378, no. 9798 (2011): 1244–1253.

Chapter 1: How the heart works

1. "Heart Facts," Cleveland Clinic, http://my.clevelandclinic.org/services/heart/heart-blood -vessels/heart-facts; Patricia Daniels, *Body: The Complete Human* (Washington, DC: National Geographic Society, 2007).

2. Lauralee Sherwood, *Human Physiology, from Cells to Systems*, 7th ed. (Boston, MA: Cengage Learning, 2010), p. 309.

3. Lauralee Sherwood, *Human Physiology, from Cells to Systems*, 8th ed. (Boston, MA: Cengage Learning, 2012), pp. 310–315.

4. Rodney A. Rhoades and David R. Bell, eds., *Medical Physiology: Principles for Clinical Medicine*, 3rd ed. (Philadelphia, PA: Lippincott Williams & Wilkins, 2009), pp. 26–27.

5. B. J. Maron and A. Pelliccia, "The Heart of Trained Athletes: Cardiac Remodeling and the Risks of Sports, Including Sudden Death," *Circulation* 114, no. 15 (2006): 1633–1644.

6. E. Patterson and B. J. Scherlag, "Decremental Conduction in the Posterior and Anterior AV Nodal Inputs," *Journal of Interventional Cardiac Electrophysiology* 7, no. 2 (October 2002): 137–148.

Chapter 2: The athlete's heart

1. Parramon's Editorial Team, *Essential Atlas of Physiology* (Hauppauge, NY: Barron's Educational Series, 2005).

2. Aaron L. Baggish and Malissa J. Wood, "Athlete's Heart and Cardiovascular Care of the Athlete: Scientific and Clinical Update," *Circulation; Contemporary Reviews in Cardiovascular Medicine,* June 13, 2011, http://circ.ahajournals.org/content/123/23/2723.

3. Reader's Digest, *The Heart and Circulatory System* (Pleasantville, NY: Reader's Digest Association, 2000).

4. Len Kravitz, "Exercise and Resting Blood Pressure," https://www.unm.edu/~lkravitz /Article%20folder/restingbp.html.

5. Regina Avraham, *The Circulatory System* (Philadelphia, PA: Chelsea House Publishers, 2000).

6. Ibid.

7. Ibid.

8. Ibid.

9. Glenn Elert, ed. (written by his students), Power of a Human Heart, http://hypertextbook .com/facts/2003/IradaMuslumova.shtml.

Chapter 3: Heart attacks, arrhythmias, and endurance athletes

1. D. Mozaffarian et al., "Physical Activity and Incidence of Atrial Fibrillation in Older Adults: The Cardiovascular Health Study," *Circulation* 118, no. 8 (2008): 800–807.

2. P. Ofman et al., "Regular Physical Activity and Risk of Atrial Fibrillation: A Systematic Review and Meta-Analysis," *Circulation: Arrhythmia and Electrophysiology* 6, no. 2 (2013): 252–256.

3. Barry Bearak, "Caballo Blanco's Last Run: The Micah True Story," *New York Times,* May 20, 2012, http://www.nytimes.com/2012/05/21/sports/caballo-blancos-last-run-the-micah-true -story.html?pagewanted=all&_r=0.

4. Justin E. Trivax and Peter A. McCullough, "Phidippides Cardiomyopathy: A Review and Case Illustration," *Clinical Cardiology* 35 (2012): 69–73.

Chapter 4: The evidence

1. H. S. Abed et al., "Effect of Weight Reduction and Cardiometabolic Risk Factor Management on Symptom Burden and Severity in Patients with Atrial Fibrillation: A Randomized Clinical Trial," *Journal of the American Medical Association* 310, no. 19 (2013): 2050–2060, https://www.ncbi.nlm.nih.gov/pubmed/24240932.

2. Jawdat Abdulla and J. R. Nielsen, "Is the Risk of Atrial Fibrillation Higher in Athletes than in the General Population? A Systematic Review and Meta-Analysis," *Europace* 11, no. 9 (2009): 1156–1159.

3. Sources for Table 4.1: J. Karjalainen et al., "Lone Atrial Fibrillation in Vigorously Exercising Middle Aged Men: Case-Control Study," *British Medical Journal* 316, no. 7147 (1998): 1784–1785; H. Heidbüchel et al., "Endurance Sports Is a Risk Factor for Atrial Fibrillation After Ablation for Atrial Flutter," *International Journal of Cardiology* 107, no. 1 (2006): 67–72; R. Elosua et al., "Sport Practice and the Risk of Lone Atrial Fibrillation: A Case-Control Study," *International Journal of Cardiology* 108, no. 3 (2006): 332–337; L. Molina et al., "Long-Term Endurance Sport Practice Increases the Incidence of Lone Atrial Fibrillation in Men: A Follow-Up Study," *Europace* 10, no. 5 (2008): 618–623; L. Mont et al., "Physical Activity, Height, and Left Atrial Size Are Independent Risk Factors for Lone Atrial Fibrillation in Middle-Aged Healthy Individuals," *Europace* 10, no. 1 (2008): 15–20; S. Baldesberger et al., "Sinus Node Disease and Arrhythmias in the Long-Term Follow-Up of Former Professional Cyclists," *European Heart Journal* 29, no. 1 (2008): 71–78.

4. M. Myrstad et al., "Increased Risk of Atrial Fibrillation Among Elderly Norwegian Men with a History of Long-Term Endurance Sport Practice," *Scandinavian Journal of Medicine & Science in Sports* 24, no. 4 (2014): e238–e244.

5. K. Andersen et al., "Risk of Arrhythmias in 52 755 Long-Distance Cross-Country Skiers: A Cohort Study," *European Heart Journal* 34, no. 47 (2013): 3624–3631.

6. M. Wilhelm et al., "Gender Differences of Atrial and Ventricular Remodeling and Autonomic Tone in Nonelite Athletes," *American Journal of Cardiology* 108, no. 10 (2011): 1489–1495.

7. I. R. Hanna et al., "The Relationship Between Stature and the Prevalence of Atrial Fibrillation in Patients with Left Ventricular Dysfunction," *Journal of the American College of Cardiology* 47, no. 8 (2006): 1683–1688.

8. Mont et al., "Physical Activity, Height, and Left Atrial Size Are Independent Risk Factors."

9. F. Van Buuren et al., "The Occurrence of Atrial Fibrillation in Former Top-Level Handball Players Above the Age of 50," *Acta Cardiologica* 67, no. 2 (2012): 213–220.

10. E. Patterson et al., "Triggered Firing in Pulmonary Veins Initiated by In Vitro Autonomic Nerve Stimulation," *HeartRhythm* 2, no. 6 (2005): 624–631.

11. E. Guasch et al., "Atrial Fibrillation Promotion by Endurance Exercise: Demonstration and Mechanistic Exploration in an Animal Model," *Journal of the American College of Cardiology* 62, no. 1 (2013): 68–77; J. R. Ruiz, M. Joyner, and A. Lucia, "CrossTalk Opposing View: Prolonged Intense Exercise Does Not Lead to Cardiac Damage," *Journal of Physiology* 591, no. 20 (2013): 4943–4945.

12. R. Aschar-Sobbi et al., "Increased Atrial Arrhythmia Susceptibility Induced by Intense Endurance Exercise in Mice Requires TNFα," *Nature Communications* 6 (2015): 6018.

13. Wilhelm et al., "Gender Differences of Atrial and Ventricular Remodeling."

14. A. Frustaci et al., "Histological Substrate of Atrial Biopsies in Patients with Lone Atrial Fibrillation," *Circulation* 96, no. 4 (1997): 1180–1184.

15. Y. Guo, G. Y. H. Lip, and S. Apostolakis, "Inflammation in Atrial Fibrillation," *Journal of the American College of Cardiology* 60, no. 22 (2012): 2263–2270.

16. M. K. Chung et al., "C-Reactive Protein Elevation in Patients with Atrial Arrhythmias: Inflammatory Mechanisms and Persistence of Atrial Fibrillation," *Circulation* 104, no. 24 (2001): 2886–2891.

17. M. Harada, D. R. Van Wagoner, and S. Nattel, "Role of Inflammation in Atrial Fibrillation Pathophysiology and Management," *Circulation Journal* 79, no. 3 (2015): 495–502.

18. D. R. Swanson, "Atrial Fibrillation in Athletes: Implicit Literature-Based Connections Suggest that Overtraining and Subsequent Inflammation May Be a Contributory Mechanism," *Medical Hypotheses* 66, no. 6 (2006): 1085–1092.

19. L. L. Smith, "Cytokine Hypothesis of Overtraining: A Physiological Adaptation to Excessive Stress?" *Medicine & Science in Sports & Exercise* 32, no. 2 (2000): 317–331.

20. M. M. Lindsay and F. G. Dunn. "Biochemical Evidence of Myocardial Fibrosis in Veteran Endurance Athletes," *British Journal of Sports Medicine* 41, no. 7 (2007): 447–452.

21. K. O'Donnell et al., "Self-Esteem Levels and Cardiovascular and Inflammatory Responses to Acute Stress," *Brain, Behavior, and Immunity* 22, no. 8 (2008): 1241–1247.

22. N. Koivula, P. Hassmén, and J. Fallby, "Self-Esteem and Perfectionism in Elite Athletes: Effects on Competitive Anxiety and Self-Confidence," *Personality and Individual Differences* 32, no. 5 (2002): 865–875.

23. A. Y. Tan and P. Zimetbaum, "Atrial Fibrillation and Atrial Fibrosis," *Journal of Cardiovascular Pharmacology* 57, no. 6 (2011): 625–629; L. Yue, J. Xie, and S. Nattel, "Molecular Determinants of Cardiac Fibroblast Electrical Function and Therapeutic Implications for Atrial Fibrillation," *Cardiovascular Research* 89, no. 4 (2011): 744–753.

24. G. Wyse et al., "Lone Atrial Fibrillation: Does It Exist?" *Journal of the American College of Cardiology* 63, no. 17 (2014): 1715–1723.

25. M. C. Wijffels et al., "Atrial Fibrillation Begets Atrial Fibrillation: A Study in Awake Chronically Instrumented Goats," *Circulation* 92, no. 7 (1995): 1954–1968.

26. M. Allessie, "The 'Second Factor': A First Step Toward Diagnosing the Substrate of Atrial Fibrillation?" *Journal of the American College of Cardiology* 53, no. 14 (2009): 1192–1193.

27. C. J. Garratt et al., "Repetitive Electrical Remodeling by Paroxysms of Atrial Fibrillation in the Goat: No Cumulative Effect on Inducibility or Stability of Atrial Fibrillation," *Journal of Cardiovascular Electrophysiology* 10, no. 8 (1999): 1101–1108; D. M. Todd et al., "Repetitive 4-Week Periods of Atrial Electrical Remodeling Promote Stability of Atrial Fibrillation: Time Course of a Second Factor Involved in the Self-Perpetuation of Atrial Fibrillation," *Circulation* 109, no. 11 (2004): 1434–1439.

28. M. K. Stiles, "Paroxysmal Lone Atrial Fibrillation Is Associated with an Abnormal Atrial Substrate: Characterizing the 'Second Factor,'" *Journal of American College of Cardiology* 53, no. 14 (2009): 1182–1191.

29. Allessie, "The 'Second Factor.'"

30. M. T. Viitasalo, R. Kala, and A. Eisalo, "Ambulatory Electrocardiographic Recording in Endurance Athletes," *British Heart Journal* 47, no. 3 (1982): 213–220.

31. J. A. Pantano and R. J. Oriel, "Prevalence and Nature of Cardiac Arrhythmias in Apparently Normal Well-Trained Runners," *American Heart Journal* 104, no. 4 (1982): 762–768; D. A. Talan et al., "Twenty-Four Hour Continuous ECG Recordings in Long-Distance Runners," *Chest* 82, no. 1 (1982): 19–24; P. Palatini et al., "Prevalence and Possible Mechanisms of Ventricular Arrhythmias in Athletes," *American Heart Journal* 110, no. 3 (1985): 560–567.

32. A. Biffi et al., "Long-Term Clinical Significance of Frequent and Complex Ventricular Tachyarrhythmias in Trained Athletes," *Journal of the American College of Cardiology* 40, no. 3 (2002): 446–452.

33. A. Biffi et al., "Impact of Physical Deconditioning on Ventricular Tachyarrhythmias in Trained Athletes," *Journal of the American College of Cardiology* 44, no. 5 (2004): 1053–1058.

34. H. Heidbüchel et al., "High Prevalence of Right Ventricular Involvement in Endurance Athletes with Ventricular Arrhythmias: Role of an Electrophysiologic Study in Risk Stratification," *European Heart Journal* 24, no. 16 (2003): 1473–1480.

35. R. Shave et al., "Exercise-Induced Cardiac Troponin Elevation: Evidence, Mechanisms, and Implications," *Journal of the American College of Cardiology* 56, no. 3 (2010): 169–176.

36. T. Eijsvogels et al., "Effect of Prolonged Walking on Cardiac Troponin Levels," *American Journal of Cardiology* 105, no. 2 (2010): 267–272; E. Serrano-Ostáriz et al., "Cardiac Biomarkers and Exercise Duration and Intensity During a Cycle-Touring Event," *Clinical Journal of Sport Medicine* 19, no. 4 (2009): 293–299; E. Serrano-Ostáriz et al., "The Impact of Exercise Duration and Intensity on the Release of Cardiac Biomarkers," *Scandinavian Journal of Medicine & Science in Sports* 21, no. 2 (2011): 244–249.

37. H. Hamasaki, "The Effects of Exercise on Natriuretic Peptides in Individuals Without Heart Failure," *Sports* 4, no. 2 (2016): 32.

38. R. Corsetti et al., "Cardiac Indexes, Cardiac Damage Biomarkers and Energy Expenditure in Professional Cyclists During the Giro d'Italia 3-Weeks Stage Race," *Biochemia Medica* 22, no 2 (2012): 237–246.

39. N. Mousavi et al., "Relation of Biomarkers and Cardiac Magnetic Resonance Imaging After Marathon Running," *American Journal of Cardiology* 103, no. 10 (2009): 1467–1472.

40. A. Urhausen et al., "Clinical Significance of Increased Cardiac Troponins T and I in Participants of Ultra-Endurance Events," *American Journal of Cardiology* 94, no. 5 (2004): 696–698.

41. T. G. Neilan et al., "Myocardial Injury and Ventricular Dysfunction Related to Training Levels Among Nonelite Participants in the Boston Marathon," *Circulation* 114, no. 22 (2006): 2325–2333.

42. A. Pelliccia et al., "Remodeling of Left Ventricular Hypertrophy in Elite Athletes After Long-Term Deconditioning," *Circulation* 105, no. 8 (2002): 944–949.

43. A. D. Elliott and A. La Gerche, "The Right Ventricle Following Prolonged Endurance Exercise: Are We Overlooking the More Important Side of the Heart? A Meta-Analysis," *British Journal of Sports Medicine* 49, no. 11 (2015): 724–729.

44. A. La Gerche et al., "Exercise-Induced Right Ventricular Dysfunction and Structural Remodelling in Endurance Athletes," *European Heart Journal* 33, no. 8 (2012): 998–1006; N. Mousavi, A. Czarnecki, K. Kumar, N. Fallah-Rad, M. Lytwyn, S. Y. Han, A. Francis, J. R. Walker, I. D. Kirkpatrick, T. G. Neilan, S. Sharma, and D. S. Jassal, "Relation of Biomarkers and Cardiac Magnetic Resonance Imaging After Marathon Running," *American Journal of Cardiology* 103 (2009): 1467–1472 .

45. M. Sanz-de la Garza et al., "Acute, Exercise Dose-Dependent Impairment in Atrial Performance During an Endurance Race: 2D Ultrasound Speckle-Tracking Strain Analysis," *Journal of the American College of Cardiology: Cardiovascular Imaging* (2016).

46. P. S. Douglas et al., "Different Effects of Prolonged Exercise on the Right and Left Ventricles," *Journal of the Amerian College of Cardiology* 15, no. 1 (1990): 64–69.

47. B. Benito et al., "Cardiac Arrhythmogenic Remodeling in a Rat Model of Long-Term Intensive Exercise Training," *Circulation* 123, no. 1 (2011): 13–22.

48. D. Corrado et al., "Does Sports Activity Enhance the Risk of Sudden Death in Adolescents and Young Adults?" *Journal of the American College of Cardiology* 42, no. 11 (2003): 1959–1963.

49. A. La Gerche et al., "Lower than Expected Desmosomal Gene Mutation Prevalence in Endurance Athletes with Complex Ventricular Arrhythmias of Right Ventricular Origin," *Heart* 96, no. 16 (2010): 1268–1274.

50. H. Heidbüchel, D. L. Prior, and A. La Gerche, "Ventricular Arrhythmias Associated with Long-Term Endurance Sports: What Is the Evidence?" *British Journal of Sports Medicine* 46, no. S1 (2012): i44–i50.

51. A. C. Sawant et al., "Exercise Has a Disproportionate Role in the Pathogenesis of Arrhythmogenic Right Ventricular Dysplasia/Cardiomyopathy in Patients Without Desmosomal Mutations," *Journal of the American Heart Association* 3, no. 6 (2014).

52. C. A. James et al., "Exercise Increases Age-Related Penetrance and Arrhythmic Risk in Arrhythmogenic Right Ventricular Dysplasia/Cardiomyopathy–Associated Desmosomal Mutation Carriers," *Journal of the American College of Cardiology* 62, no. 14 (2013): 1290–1297.

53. A. C. Sawant and H. Calkins, "Sports in Patients with Arryhthmogenic Right Ventricular Dysplasia/Cardiomyopathy and Desmosomal Mutations," *Herz* 40 (2015): 402–409.

54. C. M. Albert et al., "Triggering of Sudden Death from Cardiac Causes by Vigorous Exertion," *New England Journal of Medicine* 343, no. 19 (2000): 1355–1361.

55. T. D. Noakes et al., "Autopsy-Proved Coronary Atherosclerosis in Marathon Runners," *New England Journal of Medicine* 301, no. 2 (1979): 86–89.

56. S. Möhlenkamp et al., "Running: The Risk of Coronary Events: Prevalence and Prognostic Relevance of Coronary Atherosclerosis in Marathon Runners," *European Heart Journal* 29, no. 15 (2008): 1903–1910.

57. A. La Gerche, "The Potential Cardiotoxic Effects of Exercise," *Canadian Journal of Cardiology* 32, no. 4 (2016): 421–428.

58. S. Möhlenkamp et al., "Coronary Atherosclerosis Burden, but Not Transient Troponin Elevation, Predicts Long-Term Outcome in Recreational Marathon Runners," *Basic Research in Cardiology* 109, no. 1 (2013): 1–11

59. J. G. Schwartz et al., "Does Elite Athleticism Enhance or Inhibit Coronary Artery Plaque Formation?" *Journal of the American College of Cardiology* 55, no. A173 (2010).

60. R. Puri et al., "Impact of Statins on Serial Coronary Calcification During Atheroma Progression and Regression," *Journal of American College of Cardiology* 65, no. 13 (2015): 1273–1282.

61. La Gerche, "The Potential Cardiotoxic Effects of Exercise."

62. P. Schnohr et al., "Dose of Jogging and Long-Term Mortality: The Copenhagen City Heart Study," *Journal of the American College of Cardiology* 65, no. 5 (2015): 411–419.

63. J. H. Kim et al., "Cardiac Arrest During Long-Distance Running Races," *New England Journal of Medicine* 366, no. 2 (2012): 130–140.

Chapter 5: What to look for in yourself

1. S. C. Larsson et al., "Alcohol Consumption and Risk of Atrial Fibrillation: A Prospective Study and Dose-Response Meta-analysis," *Journal of the American College of Cardiology* 64, no. 3 (2014): 281–289; S. Kodama et al., "Alcohol Consumption and Risk of Atrial Fibrillation: A Meta-Analysis," *Journal of the American College of Cardiology* 57, no. 4 (2011): 427–436.

2. S. Dixit et al., "Consumption of Caffeinated Products and Cardiac Ectopy," *Journal of the American Heart Association* 5, no. 1 (2016): e002503.

3. D. Caldeira et al, "Caffeine Does Not Increase the Risk of Atrial Fibrillation: A Systematic Review and Meta-Analysis of Observational Studies," *Heart* 99, no. 19 (2013): 1383–1389.

4. M. Cheng et al., "Caffeine Intake and Atrial Fibrillation Incidence: Dose Response Meta-Analysis of Prospective Cohort Studies," *Canadian Journal of Cardiology* 30, no. 4 (2014): 448–454.

5. R. Lemery et al., "A Prospective Placebo Controlled Randomized Study of Caffeine in Patients with Supraventricular Tachycardia Undergoing Electrophysiologic Testing," *Journal of Cardiovascular Electrophysiology* 26, no. 1 (2015): 1–6.

6. M. Ding et al., "Long-Term Coffee Consumption and Risk of Cardiovascular Disease: A Systematic Review and a Dose-Response Meta-Analysis of Prospective Cohort Studies," *Circulation* 129, no. 6 (2014): 643–659.

7. J. A. Drezner et al., "Electrocardiographic Screening in National Collegiate Athletic Association Athletes," *American Journal of Cardiology* 118, no. 5 (2016): 754–759.

8. E. Marijon, A. Uy-Evanado, F. Dumas, N. Karam, K. Reinier, C. Teodorescu, K. Narayanan, K. Gunson, J. Jui, X. Jouven, and S. S. Chugh, "Warning Symptoms Are Associated with Survival from Sudden Cardiac Arrest," *Annals of Internal Medicine* 164, no. 1 (January 2016): 23–29.

9. J. H. Pope, et al., "Missed Diagnoses of Acute Cardiac Ischemia in the Emergency Department," *New England Journal of Medicine* 342 (2000): 1163–1170.

10. G. Chiaramonte, "Gender Bias in the Diagnosis, Treatment, and Interpretation of CHD Symptoms," Cardiovascular Research Foundation, October 12, 2008.

Chapter 7: Addicted to exertion

1. M. D. Griffiths, A. Szabó, and A. Terry, "The Exercise Addiction Inventory: A Quick and Easy Screening Tool for Health Practitioners," *British Journal of Sports Medicine* 39 (2005): e30.

2. A. Szabo, M. D. Griffiths, and Z. Demetrovics, "Exercise Addiction," in *Neuropathology of Drug Addictions and Substance Misuse,* vol. 3, edited by V. R. Preedy (London: Academic Press, 2016), 984–992.

3. Ibid.

4. Ibid.

5. Ibid.

6. Ibid.

7. K. Mónok, K. Berczik, R. Urbán, A. Szabó, M. D. Griffiths, and J. Farkas et al., "Psychometric Properties and Concurrent Validity of Two Exercise Addiction Measures: A Population Wide Study," *Psychology of Sport and Exercise* 13, no. 6 (2012): 739–746.

8. J. Youngman and D. Simpson, "Risk for Exercise Addiction: A Comparison of Triathletes Training for Sprint-, Olympic-, Half-Ironman-, and Ironman-Distance Triathlons," *Journal of Clinical Sport Psychology* 8, no. 1 (2014): 19–37.

Chapter 8: Treatment options for athlete arrhythmia

1. D. Lakkireddy, D. Atkins, J. Pillarisetti et al., "Effect of Yoga on Arrhythmia Burden, Anxiety, Depression, and Quality of Life in Paroxysmal Atrial Fibrillation: The YOGA My Heart Study," *Journal of the American College of Cardiology* 61 (2013): 1177–1182.

2. M. Wahlstrom, M. Rydell Karlsson, J. Medin, and V. Frykman, "Effects of Yoga in Patients with Paroxysmal Atrial Fibrillation—a Randomized Controlled Study," *European Journal of Cardiovascular Nursing* 14 (2016): 1–7.

3. P. Alboni et al., "Outpatient Treatment of Recent-Onset Atrial Fibrillation with the 'Pill-in-the-Pocket' Approach," *New England Journal of Medicine* 351, no. 23 (2004): 2384–2391.

4. M. Haïssaguerre et al., "Spontaneous Initiation of Atrial Fibrillation by Ectopic Beats Originating in the Pulmonary Veins," *New England Journal of Medicine* 339, no. 10 (1998): 659–666.

5. K.-H. Kuck et al., "Cryoballoon or Radiofrequency Ablation for Paroxysmal Atrial Fibrillation," *New England Journal of Medicine* 374, no. 23 (2016): 2235–2245.

6. N. Calvo et al., "Efficacy of Circumferential Pulmonary Vein Ablation of Atrial Fibrillation in Endurance Athletes," *Europace* 12, no. 1 (2010): 30–36.

7. P. Koopman et al., "Efficacy of Radiofrequency Catheter Ablation in Athletes with Atrial Fibrillation," *Europace* 13, no. 10 (2011): 1386–1393.

Chapter 9: The takeaway

1. A. R. Gaby, "The Role of Coenzyme Q10 in Clinical Medicine: Part II. Cardiovascular Disease, Hypertension, Diabetes Mellitus and Infertility," *Alternative Medicine Review* 1, no. 3 (1996): 168–175.

2. S. A. Mortensen et al., "Coenzyme Q10: Clinical Benefits with Biochemical Correlates Suggesting a Scientific Breakthrough in the Management of Chronic Heart Failure," *International Journal of Tissue Reactions* 12, no. 3 (1990): 155–162.

3. T. Fujioka, Y. Sakamoto, and G. Mimura, "Clinical Study of Cardiac Arrhythmias Using a 24-Hour Continuous Electrocardiographic Recorder (5th Report)—Antiarrhythmic Action of Coenzyme Q10 in Diabetics," *Tohoku Journal of Experimental Medicine* 141 (1983): 453–463.

4. T. Rundek et al., "Atorvastatin Decreases the Coenzyme Q10 Level in the Blood of Patients at Risk for Cardiovascular Disease and Stroke," *Archives of Neurology* 61, no. 6 (2004): 889–892.

5. P. H. Langsjoen et al., "Long-Term Efficacy and Safety of Coenzyme Q10 Therapy for Idiopathic Dilated Cardiomyopathy," *American Journal of Cardiology* 65, no. 7 (1990): 521–523.

6. E. G. Bliznakov and D. J. Wilkins, "Biochemical and Clinical Consequences of Inhibiting Coenzyme Q10 Biosynthesis by Lipid-Lowering HMG-CoA Reductase Inhibitors (Statins): A Critical Overview," *Advances in Therapy* 15, no. 4 (1998): 218–228.

7. F. L. Crane, "Biochemical Functions of Coenzyme Q10," *Journal of American College of Nutrition* 20, no. 6 (2001): 591–598.

8. R. Stocker, V. W. Bowry, and B. Frei, "Ubiquinol-10 Protects Human Low Density Lipoprotein More Efficiently Against Lipid Peroxidation than Does Alpha-Tocopherol," *Proceedings of the National Academy of Sciences* 88, no. 5 (1991): 1646–1650.

9. J. J. DiNicolantonio et al., "L-Carnitine in the Secondary Prevention of Cardiovascular Disease: Systematic Review and Meta-Analysis," *Mayo Clinic Proceedings* 88, no. 6 (2013): 544–551.

10. S. M. Marcovina et al., "Translating the Basic Knowledge of Mitochondrial Functions to Metabolic Therapy: Role of L-Carnitine," *Translational Research* 161, no. 2 (2013): 73–84.

11. R. A. Koeth et al., "Intestinal Microbiota Metabolism of L-Carnitine, a Nutrient in Red Meat, Promotes Atherosclerosis," *Nature Medicine* 19 (2013): 576–585; W. H. Wilson Tang et al., "Intestinal Microbial Metabolism of Phosphatidylcholine and Cardiovascular Risk," *New England Journal of Medicine* 368 (2013): 1575–1584.

12. J. Pekala et al., "L-Carnitine—Metabolic Functions and Meaning in Humans Life," *Current Drug Metabolism* 12, no. 7 (2011): 667–678.

13. V. U. Menon et al., "Iodine Status and Its Correlations with Age, Blood Pressure, and Thyroid Volume in South Indian Women Above 35 Years of Age (Amrita Thyroid Survey)," *Indian Journal of Endocrinology and Metabolism* 15, no. 4 (2011): 309–315.

14. D. Brownstein, *Iodine: Why You Need It, Why You Can't Live Without It,* 5th ed. (West Bloomfield, MI: Medical Alternatives Press, 2014).

15. Ibid.

16. Ibid.

17. Ibid.

18. "Iodine," Linus Pauling Institute Micronutrient Information Center, Oregon State University, March 30, 2016, http://www.lpi.oregonstate.edu/mic/minerals/iodine.

19. T. T. Zava and D. T. Zava, "Assessment of Japanese Iodine Intake Based on Seaweed Consumption in Japan: A Literature-Based Analysis," *Thyroid Research* 4, no. 14 (2011).

20. Brownstein, *Iodine.*

21. "Coronary Heart Disease Death Rate by Country," *World Health Rankings,* http://www.worldlifeexpectancy.com/cause-of-death/coronary-heart-disease/by-country/.

22. R. A. Sunde, "Selenium," in *Modern Nutrition in Health and Disease, 11th ed.,* ed. A. C. Ross et al. (Philadelphia, PA: Lippincott Williams & Wilkins, 2012), pp. 225–237.

23. "Garlic: Uses, Side Effects, Interactions and Warnings," *WebMD,* http://www.webmd.com/vitamins-supplements/ingredientmono-300-garlic.aspx?activeingredientid=300.

24. J. Y. Chan et al., "A Review of the Cardiovascular Benefits and Antioxidant Properties of Allicin," *Phytotherapy Research* 27, no. 5 (2013): 637–646.

25. S. E. Chiuve et al., "Plasma and Dietary Magnesium and Risk of Sudden Cardiac Death in Women," *American Journal of Clinical Nutrition* 93, no. 2 (2011): 253–260; L. C. Del Gobbo et al., "Circulating and Dietary Magnesium and Risk of Cardiovascular Disease: A Systematic Review and Meta-Analysis of Prospective Studies," *American Journal of Clinical Nutrition* 98, no. 1 (2013): 160–173.

26. H. Alp et al., "Protective Effects of Hawthorn (Crataegus Oxyacantha) Extract Against Digoxin-Induced Arrhythmias in Rats," *Anatolian Journal of Cardiology* 15, no. 12 (2015): 970–975; R. Tankanow et al., "Interaction Study Between Digoxin and a Preparation of Hawthorn (Crataegus Oxyacantha)," *Journal of Clinical Pharmacology* 43, no. 6 (2003): 637–642.

27. L. G. Miller, "Herbal Medicinals: Selected Clinical Considerations Focusing on Known or Potential Drug-Herb Interactions," *Archives of Internal Medicine* 158, no. 20 (1998): 2200–2211.

28. J. Hippisley-Cox and C. Coupland, "Risk of Myocardial Infarction in Patients Taking Cyclo-Oxygenase-2 Inhibitors or Conventional Non-steroidal Anti-inflammatory Drugs: Population Based Nested Case-Control Analysis," *BMJ* 330 (2005): 1366–1369; P. McGettigan and D. Henry, "Cardiovascular Risk with Non-Steroidal Anti-Inflammatory Drugs: Systematic Review of Population-Based Controlled Observational Studies," *PLoS Medicine* 8, no. 9 (2011); S. Trelle et al., "Cardiovascular Safety of Non-steroidal Anti-inflammatory Drugs: Network Meta-analysis," *BMJ* 342 (2011): 7086.

29. M. Schmidt, F. Christian Christiansen, F. Mehnert, K. Rothman, and H. Toft Sørensen, "Non-steroidal Anti-inflammatory Drug Use and Risk of Atrial Fibrillation or Flutter: Population Based Case-Control Study," *BMJ* 343 (2011).

30. B. Krijthe, J. Heeringa, A. Hofman, O. Franco, and B. Stricker, "Non-steroidal Anti-inflammatory Drugs and the Risk of Atrial Fibrillation: a Population-Based Follow-up Study," *BMJ Open* 4, no. 4 (2014).

31. J. Bradley, K. Brandt, B. Katz, L. Kalasinski, and S. Ryan, "Comparison of an Anti-inflammatory Dose of Ibuprofen, an Analgesic Dose of Ibuprofen, and Acetaminophen in the Treatment of Patients with Osteoarthritis of the Knee," *New England Journal of Medicine* 325 (1991): 87–91.

32. K. Van Wijck, K. Lenaerts, A. Van Bijnen, et al., "Aggravation of Exercise-Induced Intestinal Injury by Ibuprofen in Athletes," *Medicine & Science in Sports & Exercise* 44 (2012): 2257–2262.

33. Rachel Lampert et al., "Safety of Sports for Athletes with Implantable Cardioverter Defibrillators: Results of a Prospective Multinational Registry," *Circulation* 217 (2013): 2021–2030, http://circ.ahajournals.org/content/127/20/2021.

Epilogue

1. J. Fell and D. Williams, "The Effect of Aging on Skeletal-Muscle Recovery from Exercise: Possible Implications for Aging Athletes," *Journal of Aging and Physical Activity* 16, no. 1 (January 2008): 97–115.

GLOSSARY

Ablation: A catheter procedure to burn and kill the cells in small areas of the heart to prevent the propagation of abnormal electrical signals.

Angina pectoris: Commonly known as angina, this is the sensation of chest pain, pressure, or squeezing, often due to restricted blood supply (ischemia) of the heart muscle.

Arrhythmia: An irregular heart rhythm caused by a malfunction in the heart's electrical system.

Arrhythmogenic right ventricular cardiomyopathy (ARVC): An inherited disease of the heart muscle, sometimes called arrhythmogenic right ventricular dysplasia (ARVD). The disease is a type of nonischemic car-diomyopathy that involves primarily the right ventricle and often causes arrhythmias.

Artery: A blood vessel that carries blood away from the heart.

Asystole: Colloquially known as flatline, this is a state of no cardiac electrical activity and, therefore, no heart contractions or blood flow.

Atherosclerosis: The buildup of fats, cholesterol, and other substances in and on the artery walls.

Athlete's Heart: A nonpathological condition seen in many athletes in which the heart is enlarged and the resting heart rate is lower than average; it is a normal adaptive response to sustained exercise.

Atrial fibrillation: AF, or A-fib, is an abnormal heart rhythm characterized by rapid and irregular beating. Occasionally there may be heart palpitations, fainting, shortness of breath, or chest pain. The condition can be associated with an increased risk of heart failure, dementia, and stroke. It is a type of supraventricular tachycardia. The rate of atrial activation during AF is usually between 300 and 500 beats per minute.

Atrial flutter: An abnormal fast heart rhythm that occurs in the atria of the heart. Atrial flutter is a more organized and slightly slower rhythm than AF. The atrial rate during flutter is usually between 200 and 300 beats per minute. While this rhythm occurs most often in individuals with cardiovascular disease (e.g., hypertension, coronary artery disease, and cardiomyopathy) and diabetes mellitus, it may occur spontaneously in people with otherwise normal hearts.

Atrial tachycardia: An abnormally fast heart rhythm occurring in the atria of the heart, usually from one discrete area.

Atrioventricular (AV) node: The AV node is an area of specialized tissue between the atria and the ventricles of the heart, specifically in the posteroinferior region of the interatrial septum near the opening of the coronary sinus, which conducts the normal electrical impulse from the atria to the ventricles.

Atrium: The atrium (plural: *atria*), or auricle, is one of the two blood collection chambers of the heart. It receives blood as it returns to the heart to start a circulating cycle, whereas the ventricle pumps blood out of the heart to complete a new cycle.

Bigeminy: A descriptor for a heart arrhythmia in which there is a continuous alternation of long and short heartbeats.

Bradycardia: A slow heart rate. In adults younger than age 15, bradycardia is usually defined as a rate of less than 50 beats per minute. The lower limit of normal follows a bell curve distribution, meaning that, for some, heart rates lower than 50 are normal.

Cardiac action potential: A short-lasting event in which the membrane potential (the difference of potential between the interior and the exterior) of a cardiac cell rises and falls following a consistent trajectory.

Cardiac arrest: A sudden stop in effective blood flow due to the failure of the heart to contract effectively.

Cardiac defibrillator: A device that applies electric current (shock) to the heart to depolarize the heart muscle and terminate its arrhythmia; this allows the sinoatrial (SA) node to reestablish the normal sinus rhythm of the heart. See **Implantable cardioverter defibrillator.**

Cardiac event monitor or mobile cardiac outpatient telemetry: A portable device for continually monitoring an ECG. These devices connect with a remote monitoring station for real-time monitoring.

Cardiomyopathy: A general term for any number of diseases that affect the heart muscle.

Cardioversion: A medical procedure to convert a cardiac arrhythmia to a normal sinus rhythm using an electric shock synchronized with the heart's R wave.

Defibrillation: Restoration of the normal rhythm of a fibrillating heart (ventricular tachycardia or ventricular fibrillation) through the use of an unsynchronized electric shock.

Depolarization: A sudden and dramatic electrical change within a cell.

Diastole: The part of the cardiac cycle when the relaxed heart fills with blood following systole, or contraction.

Echocardiogram: Often referred to as a cardiac echo or simply an echo, it is a sonogram used to create images of the heart.

Electrocardiogram (ECG or EKG): A graph of voltage versus time of the electrical activity of the heart detected by electrodes in contact with the skin. See **Electrocardiography.**

Electrocardiography: The process of recording the electrical activity of the heart over a period of time using electrodes placed on the skin. The electrodes detect the tiny electrical changes on the skin that arise from the heart muscle's electrophysiologic pattern of depolarizing and repolarizing during each heartbeat. Each of the leads of a typical ECG looks at the electrical activation of the heart from a different vantage point.

Endurance events: Sports that demand a high circulation of blood and last several minutes to many hours. For the purposes of this book, we classify running, cycling, triathlon, cross-country skiing, swimming, flat-water rowing, canoeing, kayaking, and stand-up paddling as endurance events.

Fibrillation: See **Atrial fibrillation** and **Ventricular fibrillation.**

Gap junction: A specialized intercellular connection that allows charged particles to pass directly from one cardiac cell into another.

Heart attack: See **Myocardial infarction.**

His-Purkinje bundles/network: A collection of heart muscle cells specialized for electrical conduction. As part of the electrical conduction system of the heart, this network transmits the electrical impulses from the AV node and eventually to the Purkinje fibers, which provide electrical conduction to the ventricles, causing the cardiac muscle of the ventricles to contract at a paced interval.

Holter monitor: A portable device for continuously monitoring various electrical activity of the cardiovascular system via electrocardiography. It is typically worn for 24–48 hours.

Hypertrophic cardiomyopathy (HCM): An abnormal thickening of the heart's muscle, usually concentrated in the septum between the left and right ventricles. HCM usually afflicts athletes younger than age 35 and is congenital.

Implantable cardioverter defibrillator (ICD): Also called an automated implantable cardioverter defibrillator (AICD), this device is implanted inside the body in order to automatically perform, when required, cardioversion, defibrillation, and (in modern versions that include a pacemaker) pacing of the heart.

Ischemia: A restriction in blood supply to tissues, causing a shortage of oxygen and glucose needed to keep tissue alive.

Long QT syndrome: A rare, usually inherited heart condition in which delayed repolarization of the heart following a heartbeat increases the risk of episodes of torsades de pointes (a form of irregular heartbeat that originates in the ventricles).

Masters athlete: Any athlete competing in a "Masters" race category. Masters categories are age-graded in steps and generally start around age 40 in most sports.

Multifocal atrial tachycardia: Arrhythmia with multiple sites of atrial activity.

Myocardial infarction (MI): Commonly known as a heart attack, MI occurs when blood flow to a part of the heart stops, causing damage to the heart muscle.

Myocardium: The muscle cells of the heart.

Myofilament: Protein filaments that cause muscle cells to contract, as thick and thin myofilaments slide along each other.

Non-sustained ventricular tachycardia (NSVT): An episode of ventricular tachycardia of 3 or more beats at greater than 120 bpm that lasts 30 seconds or less.

Paroxysmal: A sudden recurrence or intensification of symptoms.

Paroxysmal supraventricular tachycardia (PSVT): Intermittent fast heart rate that originates above the ventricles and has abrupt onset and termination.

Phidippides cardiomyopathy: A disease of the heart caused by chronic excessive endurance exercise. It takes its name from the story of Phidippides, a young Greek messenger, who in 490 B.C. is said to have run 26.2 miles from Marathon to Athens to deliver the news of the Greek victory over the Persians, after which he collapsed and died.

Premature atrial complex (PAC, or premature atrial contraction): A relatively common event in which a cardiac contraction is initiated in either atrium by muscle cells that have gained "enhanced automaticity," rather than by the sinoatrial node, the normal heartbeat initiator. A PAC may be perceived as a "skipped beat" or felt as palpitations in the chest.

Premature ventricular complex (PVC, or premature ventricular contraction): Similar to PACs, PVCs are a relatively common event where the heartbeat is initiated in the ventricles.

Pulmonary artery hypertension: An increase in blood pressure in the pulmonary artery.

P wave: ECG wave that represents atrial activity, generated by the depolarization front as it transits the atria; see Figure 5.2.

QT interval: A measure of the time between the start of the Q wave and the end of the T wave in the heart's electrical cycle, as shown on an electrocardiogram. The QT interval represents electrical depolarization and repolarization of the ventricles. A prolonged QT interval is a marker for the potential of ventricular tachyarrhythmias like torsades de pointes and is a risk factor for sudden death.

Sarcoplasm: The material inside a muscle cell, not including the nucleus.

Sinoatrial node: Often abbreviated as "SA node," and also commonly called the sinus node, this is the normal natural pacemaker of the heart and is responsible for the initiation of the cardiac cycle, or heartbeat. It spontaneously generates an electrical impulse that, after conducting throughout the heart, causes the heart to contract.

Sinus rhythm: A rhythm of the heart in which depolarization of the cardiac cells originates at the sinoatrial (SA) node.

Sudden cardiac arrest (SCA): A sudden, unexpected loss of heart function, breathing, and consciousness. If not treated within minutes, death occurs. Cardiac arrest usually results from an electrical disturbance in the heart. (It is not the same as a heart attack.) This medical emergency requires immediate CPR or use of a defibrillator.

Sudden cardiac death (SCD): A sudden, unexpected death caused by loss of heart function (sudden cardiac arrest). It is the most common cause of natural death in the United States, responsible for about 325,000 adult deaths each year. SCD constitutes half of all heart disease deaths. See **Sudden cardiac arrest.**

Supraventricular tachycardia (SVT): An abnormally fast heart rhythm arising from improper electrical activity of the heart and originating at or above the atrioventricular node.

Systole: The part of the cardiac cycle when the ventricles contract, thus delivering blood to the lungs and body.

Tachycardia: A fast heart rate. In adults over age 15, tachycardia is usually defined as a resting heart rate of greater than 100 beats per minute. As with bradycardia, the upper limit of normal follows a bell curve distribution, meaning that, for some, resting heart rates greater than 100 are normal. Tachycardia is also normal during periods of stress, such as exercise.

Torsades de pointes: Meaning "twisting of the points," a form of irregular heartbeat that originates in the ventricles and can result in sudden cardiac death (SCD).

Trigeminy: A descriptor for PVCs that occur at intervals of two normal beats to one PVC.

Troponin: A group of three proteins (labeled C, I, and T) that regulate muscle contraction of skeletal and cardiac muscle. The presence of troponin in the blood system is an indicator of cardiac cell damage (e.g., heart attack).

Vein: A blood vessel that carries blood from the tissues to the heart.

Ventricle: One of two large lower chambers of the heart. Each ventricle collects and expels blood received from an atrium. The right ventricle collects deoxygenated blood from the atrium above it and pumps it into the lungs; the left ventricle pumps oxygenated blood into the body through the aorta.

Ventricular fibrillation: V-fib, or VF, is an arrhythmia in which there is uncoordinated contraction of the cardiac muscle of the ventricles due to very rapid electrical activation. Because of the lack of coordinated contraction, there is no significant cardiac output, which leads to cardiac arrest. VF is the most commonly identified arrhythmia in cardiac arrest patients.

Ventricular tachycardia: Like atrial tachycardia, VT usually originates from a discrete focus within the ventricles. When associated with accompanying heart disease, VT can be life-threatening.

Voltage-gated ion channel: A channel for ions in the cell membrane that opens and closes in response to changes in electrical potential across the membrane.

Wolff-Parkinson-White Syndrome: A disorder of the electrical system of the heart that is commonly referred to as a pre-excitation syndrome. It is caused by the presence of an abnormal conduction pathway between the heart's atria and ventricles.

INDEX

ABOUT THE AUTHORS

Chris Case is the managing editor of *VeloNews* and author of the ground-breaking article "Cycling to Extremes" that brought the problem of the athlete's heart to national attention. A neuroscience graduate of Colgate University, Case conducted clinical research at the National Institute of Mental Health in Bethesda, Maryland, and at the University of Colorado Health Sciences Center before earning his master's degree in journalism from the University of Texas at Austin. A competitive runner from the age of 12, Case rediscovered cycling in graduate school. He is a silver medalist at the US National Cyclocross Championships and Masters World Championships.

John Mandrola, MD, is a cardiac electrophysiologist as well as a runner, cyclist, and bicycle commuter. His medical practice encompasses catheter ablation, including two decades of experience with AF ablation and cardiac device implantation. He is the chief cardiology correspondent for Medscape, contributing a weekly column, journal review podcast, and interviews with academic leaders. He has been an invited speaker on multiple continents. In recent years, Mandrola has coauthored academic journal articles in the fields of electrophysiology, sports cardiology, palliative care, and outcomes research. He maintains a health, fitness, and medicine blog at www.drjohnm.org. He completed his medical training in internal medicine, cardiology, and electrophysiology at Indiana University.

Lennard Zinn is a lifelong endurance athlete and a former member of the US national cycling team whose personal story of multifocal atrial tachycardia inspired this book. He holds a degree in physics from Colorado College and has held research positions at Los Alamos National Laboratory. Zinn is the senior technical writer for *VeloNews* and has reported on major stories for the magazine for more than 30 years. Since 1982, Zinn has owned the custom bicycle-building business Zinn Cycles, Inc. He is the best-selling author of *Zinn and the Art of Road Bike Maintenance* and *Zinn and the Art of Mountain Bike Maintenance,* among other cycling titles.